—with— CHANGE

Focus on Retirement

**Resource materials for
mid-life and pre-retirement
programmes**

by
Allin Coleman
and
Anthony Chiva

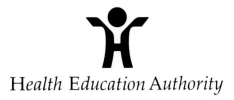

Health Education Authority

The Centre for Health and Retirement Education was
funded by the Health Education Authority. The
development and testing of these resource materials
formed a substantial part of the CHRE's programme
from 1987 to 1990.

Published by the Health Education Authority
Hamilton House
Mabledon Place
London WC1 9TX

Typeset by DP Photosetting, Aylesbury, Bucks
Printed by
Biddles Ltd, Guildford

ISBN 1 85448 182 7

Contents

Acknowledgements

On behalf of the Centre for Health and Retirement
Education, we should like to thank all the people who have
worked with us on these resource materials as administrators,
trainers, tutors and members of our Advisory Committee.

On the Advisory Committee: David Armstrong (Chair,
Centre for Extra-Mural Studies, University of London),
Sherry Clift (Bassetlaw District Health Authority), Peter
Gardonyi (Health Education Authority), Eric George (Trades
Union Congress), Brian Groombridge (Institute of
Education, University of London), Sarah Grylls (Workers'
Educational Association, Oxford), John Harte (Royal College
of General Practitioners), Jim O'Malley (Pre-Retirement
Association), Cathy Lowe (Health Education Authority), John
Saunders (Bank of England), Pam Shakespeare (Open
University) and Jo Walker (Pre-Retirement Association).

In the National Health Service Pilot Programme:
Canterbury and Thanet Health Authority (Ann Leese, Colin
Ryder and Pat Worsfold); East Cumbria Health Authority
(Ann Barlow, Francis Cunning and Geoff Pitt); East Dyfed
Health Authority (David Evans, Meiler Harries and Kevin
Tribble); Lewisham and North Southwark Health Authority
(Miriam McDaniel and Colette McGill); Pembrokeshire
Health Authority (Yvonne Johnson); Winchester Health
Authority (Mary Linton and Audrey Payne). Our thanks also
go to the senior officers within these Health Authorities who
supported this programme; to the Age Well Case Studies
Project; and to Central Nottinghamshire Health Authority for
their initial exploratory work.

In the Training Associates Programmes: Westminster
Adult Education Institute (Peter Convery, Ruth Crossick and
Robin Webster); Fareham and Gosport Institute of Adult
Education, Youth and Community Services (Julian Noble);
Newark Technical College (Saskia Mills); Brentwood Adult

Education Centre (Roy Grier and Freda Newberry); Chelmsford Adult Education Centre (Ann Bell and Jean Pitt); Essex Education Authority (David Hollins and Reg Smith).

We should also like to thank other supporting Education Authorities and all those people who participated on our pilot courses, sharing the experience with us and contributing much to the present shape of the model programme.

Joy Groombridge edited the resource materials for publication in this form. Kathy Meade, CHRE Development Officer, gave the project valuable advice and support over the two years in which she worked for the Centre. Jane Hardy and Barbara Waller patiently typed and retyped the many versions of the text.

Grateful acknowledgement is also due to Methuen and Co, Publishers for permission to reproduce on page 40 the figure and text from *Life-Span Development* by Leonie Sugarman.

ALLIN COLEMAN
HEA Pre-retirement Project Director 1982–85 and
CHRE Coordinator until his retirement in 1988.
Subsequently Consultant and part-time development officer.

ANTHONY CHIVA
CHRE Coordinator from 1988

Introduction

These resource materials are intended for use by

- personnel officers and others within organisations providing opportunities for their own employees to prepare for retirement
- consultants who make it their business to put together 'preparation for retirement packages' for employers
- tutors in adult education who put on courses either specifically for employees of one organisation or for members of the general public.

They also have a wider application in programmes concerned with mid and later life planning: in helping people to take stock and prepare for change at other life stages.

In Part One: Notes for Tutors (page 1) we explain how and why the materials were developed, and how we intend them to be used. As the programme suggested here is not information-based, but draws on a range of teaching skills, we have included in this section some hints for the less experienced tutor who may feel diffident about approaching an unfamiliar situation. The CHRE is based in a centre for adult learning at a university, and so we have found it appropriate to call the man or woman leading the group 'tutor' throughout, and the people attending 'participants'.

Part Two: The Coping with Change Model in Action (page 27) outlines a complete programme and shows how it can be adapted to suit a variety of circumstances.

We have indicated, in Appendix 1: Notes on Marketing (page 117), some ways in which such a programme may be promoted to employers, to heads of adult education centres and to people who are themselves approaching this challenging and exciting new time in their lives. Finally, Appendix 2 (page 126) looks at some of the ways in which the work may be developed.

Part One: Notes for Tutors

The Case for Change

The emphasis of this Coping with Change model for pre-retirement education is on gaining insight, not on accumulating information. It provides a practical framework in which participants can identify their experiences of change and transition in life and focus on their needs concerning another change – called retirement. The intention is to help both individuals and groups:

- to analyse their understanding of change and transition
- to explore their feelings and reactions to change
- to identify the key issues of their retirement
- to consider their choices and options
- to assess their skills and the resources available to them to put their plans into action.

Education and Retirement

The idea that it might be a good thing for people to come together in an educational environment actively to prepare for retirement has gained ground steadily since the 1950s. The earliest recorded pre-retirement course took place in the United States in 1949, and in Britain the National Old People's Welfare Council (now Age Concern) set up a Preparation for Retirement Study Group in 1955, and ran an experimental weekend residential course in 1958.

From this beginning, 'preparation for retirement' has been seen as a form of 'course'. This institutionalising of pre-retirement education brought with it two attendant problems. The first was that 'retirement', unlike any other phase in life, was being segregated from other life processes (such as becoming an adult, or becoming a parent) primarily because of its very specific associations with male employment and ageing. The second was that any educational programme requires a body of knowledge from which an appropriate scheme of study can be developed. This did not exist. A curriculum emerged by way of adoption of the concept of a hierarchy of human needs culminating in personal fulfilment, influenced by the work of the American psychologist Abraham Maslow. These human needs were identified as: good health, adequate income, accommodation, congenial associates, absorbing interests and an adequate personal philosophy of life.

Why 'Change'?

In the 1980s both the content and the methodology of pre-retirement education came under scrutiny.

In *Preparation for Retirement in England and Wales* (NIACE, 1982) Allin Coleman showed how inadequate provision of pre-retirement education was, and listed six areas of pre-retirement education which he thought needed more consideration:

1. Conceptual understanding of retirement.
2. Understanding of the aims and objectives of pre-retirement course provision.
3. Awareness of the individual needs of course members.
4. Use of the course members' experience (that vast reservoir of human resources).
5. Appropriate timing or phasing of preparation for retirement.
6. Women, as paid workers or as partners in retirement.

The report also recognised the distinctive nature of pre-retirement education, interacting as it did between the boundaries of paid employment, education and leisure.

The Impact of Pre-Retirement Education by C. Phillipson and L. Strang (University of Keele, 1983) listed some 18 recommendations for good practice in pre-retirement education. Its overall findings indicated that there was little evidence that present courses were effective. It forecast a bleak outlook for pre-retirement education unless courses reflected the changing attitudes of people to retirement, and unless the methods used became more appropriate to mature adults.

Meanwhile, Stanley Parker, working for the OPCS, produced a report, *Older Workers and Retirement* (HMSO, 1980). This included a series of statistics on workers' attitudes to work and retirement, and also put forward a helpful analysis of retirement as an event, a process and as a phase in life.

From another perspective, a number of sociologists and psychologists had been developing some valuable insights into the nature of change in human experience. In Parker's terms, many forms of intervention around retirement concentrate on the event, often linking it with a ceremony such as a retirement party. However, the actual *process* of retirement may well have begun much earlier, and it is during the process period that various forms of support (such as a pre-retirement course) may most usefully offer help to the individual to prepare for the changes to be experienced in the foreseeable future.

In *Bereavement: Studies of Grief in Adult Life* (Tavistock, 1972) Colin Murray Parkes showed that when people identified change as *gain* the period of transition was quite smooth, though not necessarily short, and often resulted in personal development. However, when people perceived change as *loss* or even as 'a mixed blessing' they tended to resist the experience of transition. He concluded: 'resistance to change, the reluctance to give up possessions, people, status, expectations – this, I believe, is the basis of grief.' Continued unwillingness to look at the problems (if perceived as such) occasioned by any given change will not only perpetuate them, but will also lead to opportunities inherent in the situation being missed.

In *Transition: Understanding and Managing Personal Change* (Martin Robertson, 1976) B. Hopson and J. Adams identified two tasks which each individual has to undertake if a transition is to be successfully accomplished: taking control or managing the stress; understanding the process and acquiring the necessary knowledge to manage change.

During the 'process' period of retirement, the transition from paid employment, a pre-retirement course may help individuals to prepare for the changes to be experienced in the foreseeable future. The 'themes of change' which may then emerge to form the content of a pre-retirement course will certainly embrace some of the following: changes relating to concepts of self, self-esteem and role shifts; relationships and social networks; the management of time; budgeting and finance. The expert-dominated information-based series of discrete sessions no longer seems appropriate. A more integrated participant-centred learning environment is better suited to addressing Hopson and Adams's 'two tasks'. This means that tutors need to think carefully about the methods they use. Adults are highly selective about what they wish to learn and respond positively to being asked to contribute to the programme. Tutors need also to remember that adults have a range of experience which they are usually willing to share.

Development of the Model

In recent years the Health Education Authority, as part of its Health in Old Age Programme, has shown particular interest in the health issues of the pre-retirement age group, funding first the Pre-Retirement Project at the Department of Extra-Mural Studies, University of London (1982–1985) and subsequently the Centre for Health and Retirement Education (from 1986).

The Pre-Retirement Project had two main features. The first focused on the extent of pre-retirement provision for staff in the National Health Service, and the level of training given to those responsible for this work. This national survey confirmed that, although there was an agreed policy for pre-retirement education, the actual 'take-up' was low, and there was no uniform designation to any department for that service, with the result that professional groups such as health education (promotion) officers, many of whom had initial training in educational methodology, were either marginally involved or not involved at all. A report of this survey was published in 1984 and in the same year a special training 'option' on pre-retirement education was included in the annual summer school programme for health education officers at York University.

The second and complementary study was a response by the then Health Education Council (HEC) to the criticisms, particularly in the Phillipson and Strang report, of the educational relevance of many of the health sessions in pre-retirement courses. An action research programme was set up to develop more appropriate content and methodology, and involved doctors, health education officers and dieticians in particular. Two publications subsequently emerged from this work: *A Doctor's Perspective* summarised the experimental work undertaken specifically with doctors, both in private practice and in industry; *An Ideas and Resources Pack for Health Educators* brought together the results of the work with a variety of health professionals throughout the country and indicated ways in which a multi-disciplinary approach, combined with educational methods appropriate for adults, represented a major step forward in this work.

The work of the CHRE has built on both Stanley Parker's analysis and the work of Hopson and others, and concentrated on the relationship between health and retirement, between this period of transition and well-being in later life. The Coping with Change model of pre-retirement education has been developed out of these areas (see Figure 1).

A commission to replace the HEC pamphlet on health and retirement by a new booklet, *What Next? – Focus on Health*, enabled the CHRE to incorporate much of the experience from its action-research programmes and, in particular, to look at retirement as one of life's major changes, and the role of the individual in managing or coping with this change.

Over a period of three years, experimental tutor-training courses using the Coping with Change model were arranged with Lancashire Education Authority, the University of London and the Pre-Retirement Association at Holly Royde Residential Centre, University of Manchester. These helped both to create a climate for change in the approach to pre-retirement education and also underlined the unquestionable need for a national programme of training for this expanding area of work.

In 1988 the Department of Extra-Mural Studies, University of London, in collaboration with the CHRE, set

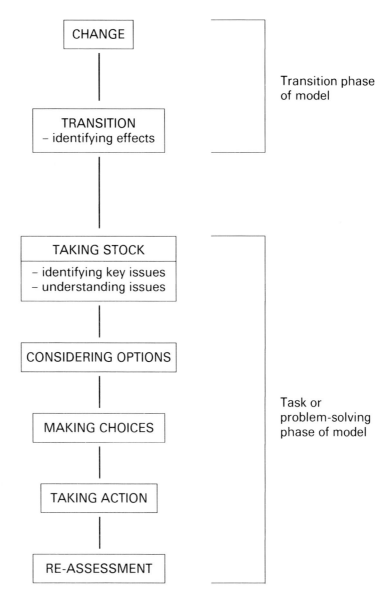

Figure 1 *Coping with Change Model*

up a new part-time diploma course in mid and later life planning. The underlying aims of this course were to promote the development of human potential in the second half of life and to encourage its maximum quality. While this diploma course presented an opportunity for people within reach of London to attend, it needs to be replicated by many other agencies to have any noticeable impact nationally. The CHRE has initiated discussions with appropriate examination boards and other bodies to explore routes for accreditation for pre-retirement education tutors in education institutions close to their homes or places of work.

Testing and Refining the Model

On the basis of three years' practical experience of developing the model in different locations and among different groups, the CHRE set out on an ambitious programme of testing and refining the model in the field. Support was canvassed from two particular sectors and professional groups.

The first group of practising pre-retirement tutors was identified in District or Regional Health Authorities. They received a short course of intensive training and supervision from the staff of the CHRE, which included systematic evaluation both of their training programmes and of their subsequent experiences in using this model. This group consisted of personnel and welfare officers, trainers, health promotion officers, nurse tutors, nursing officers and pensions staff, which indicates the extent and variety of pre-retirement education within the National Health Service. None of the group was engaged solely on pre-retirement work, which was generally considered to occupy only a small proportion of general duties with small budgets and little support or recognised systems of evaluation.

The second group, experienced in staff development, formed the CHRE's Training Associates Programme and was identified within the national system of adult education in local authority owned colleges or institutes. This group had two main tasks: (1) to train and supervise pre-retirement tutors in the use of the Coping with Change model and (2) to assist in the refining of the model from their experiences of supervising others and from the experiences of their tutors working with pre-retirement groups. The work of the Training Associates Programme in developing these resource materials was intended to be a significant step in the process towards accreditation.

We were aware that all those engaged with the CHRE in testing and refining the model came from a number of disciplines or specialist subject areas, each with particular knowledge and/or skills not necessarily directly related to pre-retirement education. This was its strength (and challenge) for the composition of both groups mirrored the national picture described by Coleman in his 1982 survey.

We were also particularly conscious that tutors would expect to receive a 'set' curriculum on which they could base their own pre-retirement courses. But the Coping with Change model was presented as a 'process' rather than a 'content' model and, as such, challenged tutors to consider fundamental questions about this area of work, such as 'Why are we doing it?', 'When are we offering it?', 'To whom are we offering it?', 'What are we offering?' and 'How do we do (or present) it?' The notion of a predetermined curriculum came under scrutiny and the possibility of developing relevant curricula to meet the needs of different or specific groups, through the process of engaging the participants themselves in articulating their own 'agenda', came to the fore.

It was clear that tutors needed to be familiar with a range of adult education teaching methods if they were to feel confident in their ability to operate the model successfully. The next section of these resource materials therefore consists of a brief outline on methodology, taken from the CHRE's own *Ideas and Resources Pack for Health Educators*, and some more detailed notes on particular techniques used are indicated in the text.

Adults Learning

How Adults Learn

For many adults approaching retirement, the invitation to attend a pre-retirement course may bring back memories of school half a century ago. If schooldays were not the happiest days of their lives, some may be suspicious of attending a course and of 'education'. Most will come with a well-developed set of expectations. They will have expectations of how the 'teacher' will proceed and of how they will be expected to react to being 'taught'. If the course programme contains a list of 'subjects' and speakers this will reinforce those expectations. If the programme mentions the word 'discussion', this is at least a hint that the course is not going to be all lecturing. Initially this too may cause some apprehension and should be explained by the course tutor/ leader as early as possible. For times have changed and, since the generation now approaching retirement started school, much research has been done into learning methods. It is becoming increasingly clear from the growing body of knowledge about how adults learn that more emphasis should be placed on the value of the period of reflection in the learning process and on the wealth of experience which adults have gained. This has implications for the course process. Within the overall design of a course, time needs to be given for reflection. Methods commonly used in the teaching of children and adolescents are not always appropriate with adults. Adults learn better from tutors who treat them as *adults*, and who assume that the mature adult:

- is highly selective about what to learn
- has a wide range of experience which is a rich resource for learning
- is willing to share both knowledge and experience and demonstrate skills with others
- is a more self-directed person than a child and responds more readily to an environment in which time is given for consultation.

It used to be thought that the older you were, the less likely you were to be able to learn anything new. The folklore held that 'you can't teach an old dog new tricks'. Psychologists and others generally assumed that both physical and mental maturation occurred at some stage in the mid-20s, after which a process of deterioration got under way. Habits may die hard

– it is in the nature of their biological function to do so – but studies into the learning abilities of adults establish that, though there may be problems with learning, adults are capable of learning new things at any age.

A learning process is the sum total of the stages which it is necessary to go through in order to acquire new knowledge, a skill or a change in attitude or behaviour. It can be set out in diagrammatic form.

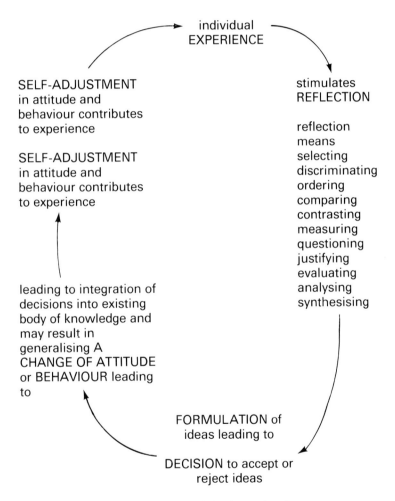

Figure 2   *A Model of the Learning Process*

Example

I receive the following information:

● it is a healthy exercise to walk for 30 minutes twice weekly, maintaining a raised pulse rate, and probably burning up about 150 calories.

I reflect upon it, and analyse it:

What are the good points about brisk walking I already know?

- fresh air
- helps fitness
- helps co-ordination
- relaxing
- it is easy – no dressing up or undressing
- it is cheap
- it can be done alone or involve the family or friends.

What are the points about brisk walking I do not know?

- what is a raised pulse rate?

I check.

- go back to the source for more information about raised pulse rate
- discover that the least complicated (subjective) method of assessment of raised pulse rate is that it accompanies being a little out of breath. The objective method is to take one's own pulse rate – this can be learned
- *either* confirm mutual trust and respect towards the source of the information *or* reject the information.

I decide

- to accept or reject the idea of walking briskly for 30 minutes twice weekly on results of *reflection* and trust in the authority of the information given.

I act

- either positively or negatively
- if positively, a feeling of conviction leads to a change which contributes to *experience*.

I evaluate the new knowledge, perhaps at some time in the future. For example, the benefits of the learning experience may include:

- confirmation of my already held views on the benefts of walking briskly
- a conscious feeling of relaxation
- a knowledge of how to check my pulse rate
- a feeling of well-being

> • confidence in any information which may come from the same source in the future.

The Tutor and the Group

In preparing to help older adults learn – from their own experience as well as from each other and from specialists – tutors need to think about their own style as 'teachers'; about the needs and interests of the course members; and about what has to be learned. Most people teach as they themselves were taught and need to ask themselves:

- Was that a good model to imitate?
- Was it too formal, prescriptive, authoritarian?
- Was it too informal and unstructured?
- Did our tutors talk too much? Too little? Too inaudibly?
- Was it relevant?

A good tutor

- exposes group participants to new possibilities for self-fulfilment
- helps them to clarify their own aspirations
- helps them to diagnose the issues which interest or concern them
- helps learners to identify life problems resulting from their learning needs
- provides physical conditions conducive to adult learning
- accepts and treats adults as people
- seeks to build relationships of trust and co-operation between the participants
- becomes a co-learner in the spirit of mutual enquiry
- involves them in a mutual process of formulating learning objectives
- shares with them the most appropriate methods to achieve those objectives
- helps them to organise themselves to undertake their tasks
- helps them to exploit their own experiences as learning resources
- gears presentation of his or her own resources to the levels of the learners' experiences
- helps them to integrate new learning into their own experiences
- involves them in devising criteria and methods to measure progress
- helps them to develop and apply self-evaluation procedures to monitor their own and the group's progress.

A good group

- encourages involvement and participation
- provides an efficient means for decision-making
- provides a forum for ideas, experiences and skills to be shared

- provides a 'safe' setting for those who are shy or reluctant to voice their opinions in public
- encourages socialising, friendship, respect for the opinions of others and mutual enjoyment
- enables members to learn consciously or sub-consciously about group behaviour and therefore about their own behaviour in a group
- helps to increase members' confidence in day-to-day working both in and away from the group
- is the reservoir of resources of all the members which is greater than the resources possessed by any single member.

Methods to Use

Learning can occur in a variety of ways; for example, when an individual is being taught, being talked at, looking or observing, engaging in discussion or learning from books. There are perhaps ten key factors which the tutor should consider in deciding on the most appropriate method:

1. Are your objectives clear?
2. Is the environment conducive to the method?
3. Is the size of the group compatible with the method?
4. Do all the members know what is expected of them?
5. If handout materials are to be used, are they readily available and in the right quantity?
6. Can sufficient time be allocated for each stage?
7. Is the material too difficult or too easy for the members?
8. Will you appoint sub-group leaders or will sub-groups appoint their own?
9. Will you have the opportunity to explain your methods to the sub-group leaders?
10. Is there to be any feedback or evaluation?

Discussion

Discussion is a natural method of exchanging information. It goes on all the time, at home, at work, in the pub or over the garden fence. But in the educational setting discussion can be used more deliberately, as when a group of people (with or without a leader) are encouraged to learn in a co-operative manner more about something they are interested in by pooling their opinions, ideas and knowledge. Discussion is more heightened, more structured than ordinary conversation.

Why use discussion?

- It is the prime example of participatory learning.
- It encourages respect for each member's point of view.
- It can be mentally stimulating and challenging for the participants.
- It focuses the minds of the group members on a common search for meanings.

- It can be an enjoyable journey of discovery for members as they measure and extend their individual knowledge.
- It enables opinions and prejudices to be challenged and/or justified.
- It maximises human contact and personal involvement within the group.
- It usually has a time limit which should reflect what can reasonably be expected from a group working together.
- It encourages listening skills.
- It encourages clear and logical speech which can readily be understood by the rest of the group.
- It represents a completely different approach to the authoritarian specialist armed with all the right answers.
- It can be an excellent way to define, analyse and produce decisions in problem-solving exercises.

The discussion method can profitably be used on almost any occasion where the agreed aim is to involve the members in the learning process. Many pre-retirement courses are advertised as discussion-based, but are really lectures with some time allowed for a question and answer period. While it is acknowledged that a great deal of informal learning through discussion goes on during the course, it is important to emphasise that 'discussion' and 'question and answer' are not the same methods of imparting information. Both techniques rely on audience (group) participation, and both need skilful handling by whoever is running the session.

Discussion in small groups can either be led or leaderless. It is advisable to use the leaderless method only with very small groups of, say, two or three people, especially if the main purpose is to gain opinions quickly, and the time is limited. In other words, it allows you to test and gather a whole variety of opinions from the group more effectively than trying to do it yourself from 'the front'.

It is more appropriate to have a leader when the main purpose is actively to engage the group in their own learning process and/or draw conclusions from known material, such as a case study.

Case study work

In pre-retirement education a case study is used simply as a teaching/learning aid, which enables group members to relate to each other and to the issues involved. It can be a particularly good method for the experienced tutor without specialist knowledge. The case study can be a story, real or fictional (or part of each), which can be related in a number of ways. It is usually written to be read but can be spoken or acted 'live' or recorded on sound or video tape. Studying the case enables group members to acquire knowledge, compare attitudes and share insights into general issues.

Reasons for using a case study

- It can introduce an element of realism into learning. It is possible for members to analyse situations that might actually occur. People can become impatient if what they are being told is too remote from their real life experiences.
- It arouses the interest of group members and gives opportunity to think through the issues.
- It deals with specific events or facts and avoids generalities.
- It encourages the adoption or interpretation of socially accepted principles to a particular circumstance.
- It provides an opportunity to work co-operatively, which establishes an atmosphere of give-and-take between the members.
- It can be used in small groups of mixed ability, with or without an elected leader, where members start off on an equal footing.
- It enables members to give their own opinions and defend them, while at the same time recognising that others in the group may have information and opinions which may lead to changes in (or reinforcement of) previously held attitudes on particular issues.
- It enables members to become conscious of their own hidden talents (or limitations) in arriving at decisions.
- It enables members to recognise that people differ in the way they view events or tackle problems. There may be more than one valid solution.
- It enables members to realise that other people may experience difficulty in resolving some of the issues in the case study.
- It develops communication skills in listening to others and in conveying ideas clearly without lengthy explanations.
- It helps to bring about a better understanding of human behaviour.
- Members often 'see' themselves, or others close to them, in situations similar to those described in the case study. Sharing in the analysis of the problems enables them to see more clearly the options available to them in real life.
- It is a flexible aid to learning.
- It enables people to talk about their feelings and attitudes without being personal.

Possible drawbacks

- Group members may feel put out at being expected to do the thinking.
- The amount of information given will never suit everybody. Time can be wasted by those who feel they cannot make decisions without having more information available.
- Members do not actually have to take responsibility for the decisions they make. Sometimes this results in a tendency

to oversimplify or to come up with way-out solutions inappropriate to the case itself.

- In a brief case study it is impossible to convey the subtle overtones of human behaviour or the succession of interactions which play a crucial part in experiences in real life.
- It can be a waste of time if not properly prepared and presented.
- Special skills are required of the leader, especially to keep the group focused on the assignment and to refrain from imposing personal views as a means of influencing group decisions.

Trigger videos

The video cassette is a relatively new educational tool and its use is well worth considering:

- It is from the eye that the brain receives more than two-thirds of its information and the video, like television, demands visual attention.
- The video has obvious relevance to real life.
- The opinions expressed invite response and provide a focus for discussion.
- Some videos are specifically designed for a pre-retirement course and are intended to help the leader and group to achieve their objectives.
- They promote understanding of the feelings, opinions and attitudes of others with which group members can readily identify.
- They are particularly useful with small groups as they encourage co-operation among group members rather than competition.
- They encourage personal anecdotal responses, an indication that in any group of mature adults each individual can draw upon a reservoir of experiences for the benefit of all members.

Other possibilities

Brainstorming is a method used to draw from the group as many ideas as possible relating to a particular area of interest or field of study. List the ideas in a prominent place as they are called out. Participants are not obliged or put under any kind of pressure to contribute. The key person is the leader who maintains the momentum of the exercise and encourages the flow of as many ideas as possible. Keep it lively by keeping it short – no evaluative comments at this stage. Normally this exercise should not exceed ten minutes. Then group members, with the help of the leader, shortlist the ideas, place them into categories or list them in order of priority, possibly holding in reserve those with less immediate relevance.

Buzz grouping is a device for dividing up a large group into smaller sub-groups (usually with a maximum of eight members) for a limited period. It enables the members to focus on one single topic. It can be used on more than one occasion during the same session with different or partly changed sub-groups. It can be used effectively in decision-making, in gaining opinions, and more generally in helping to involve shy, inarticulate or awkward members.

There may or may not be an appointed sub-group leader, depending on whether feedback is required.

How to Use the Resource Materials

An Outline of the Course Material

The resource materials are divided into sections (see Fig. 3 on page 20) which, it must be emphasised, should not necessarily be equated with the sessions of a pre-retirement course. In Stages 1–4 participants are encouraged to talk about what retirement means to them and to place this in a wider context of life in the 1990s. Next, in Stages 5–7, participants are given the opportunity to consider how they have been affected by different events in their lives, and how they have coped with or managed previous changes. In Stages 8 and 9 they identify the principal changes they anticipate retirement will bring to their lives and decide which to examine in detail. From this point the order of the course material cannot be predicted, but our experience shows that in the majority of groups four major 'themes of change' are almost always identified. Alternative treatments are suggested for issues around changes in the use of time, in financial status, in health and in personal relationships. Stages 10–12 offer participants the opportunity to consider and evaluate what they have learned.

Adapting the Material to Suit Your Programme

We believe that retirement is one of life's experiences of change, and that planning or preparing for it should begin early in one's career. The programme outlined here can be seen as part of a continuing development process. During the action research undertaken in piloting these materials, a number of alternative arrangements were made in relation to both the choice and the length of sessions. We cannot make assumptions about the precise length and number of sessions available for any particular retirement programme: much will depend on its nature. However, the most frequent formats are as follows (see Figures 4–6):

1. short non-residential courses over two to three days
2. regular meetings over six or eight weeks
3. short residential courses, often over a weekend.

Other variables are noted in the 'Options' paragraph of each section.

The most important factor is that enough time is allowed for participants to understand and harness their experience and apply their problem-solving skills to issues they see as important.

As we have indicated, the pre-retirement course outlined here is a process model. In the treatment of the themes, the

Stages

THE MEANING OF RETIREMENT

1. Getting started
2. Getting to know you
3. What does retirement mean to you?
4. Social and economic context

LOOKING AT LIFE'S CHANGES

5. Understanding change
6. The process of transition
7. Letting go and looking ahead

PREPARING FOR CHANGE

8. Retirement and change
9. Identifying themes of change

THEMES OF CHANGE – ALTERNATIVE TREATMENTS

Topics

Time

A. Transition and time
B. Analysis and use of time

Finance

A. Experience of financial change
B. Personal finance

Health

A. Health – what is it?
B. Health: taking charge

Relationships

A. Transition and relationships
B. Changing relationships

REVIEW – THE FINAL SESSION

10. Review
11. Evaluation
12. What next?

HANDOUT SHEETS

Figure 3   *An Outline of the Resource Materials*

Option One – a Two-Day Course

Advance Notice	Day One	Day Two
Letter to participants 2–3 weeks before programme begins inviting them to consider 'What does 'retirement' mean to you?' Information received is collated for participants.	The Meaning of Retirement – Stages 1–4 Looking at Life Changes – Stages 5 and 6	Selected First Theme – Topic B Selected Second Theme – Topic A
	Lunch	Lunch
	Looking at Life Changes – Stage 7 Preparing for Change – Stages 8 and 9 Selected First Theme Topic A	Selected Second Theme – Topic B Final Session – Stages 10–12

Option Two – a Two and a Half Day Course

Day One	Day Two	Day Three
The Meaning of Retirement – Stages 1–4 Looking at Life Changes – Stage 5	Looking at Life Changes – Stages 6 and 7 Preparing for Changes – Stages 8 and 9	Selected Second Theme – Topic B Selected Third Theme – Topic A
	Lunch	Lunch
	Selected First Theme – Topics A and B Selected Second Theme – Topic A	Selected Third Theme – Topic B Final Session – Stages 10–12

(*Note:* Day One is a half-day session 2–3 weeks before remaining two days)

Figure 4 *Short Two–Three Day Non-Residential Course: Two Suggested Outlines*

Half-Days		
One	**Two**	**Three**
The Meaning of Retirement – Stages 1–4 Looking at Life Changes – Stage 5	Looking at Life Changes – Stages 6 and 7 Preparing for Change – Stages 8 and 9	Selected First Theme

Four	**Five**	**Six**
Selected Second Theme	Selected Third Theme	Selected Fourth Theme Final Session – Stages 10–12

(*Note:* It is assumed that a session is three hours including a break.)

Figure 5   *Regular Meetings Over Six–Eight Sessions: Suggested Outline*

Day One	Day Two	Day Three
	Looking at Life Changes – Stages 6 and 7 Preparing for Changes – Stages 8 and 9	Selected Third Theme – Topic B Final Session – Stages 10–12
	Lunch	Lunch
	Selected First Theme – Topics A and B Selected Second Theme – Topic A	
Supper/Buffet	Supper/Buffet	
The Meaning of Retirement – Stages 1–4 Looking at Life Changes – Stage 5	Selected Second Theme – Topic B Selected Third Theme – Topic A	

(*Note*: It is assumed that a session is three hours including a break.)

Figure 6   *Short Residential Course, Often Over a Weekend: Suggested Outline*

topics and activities suggested move through the same sequence of steps (see Figure 1, page 7). Tutors should be aware that omitting a whole stage may considerably reduce the 'growth and development' potential of the programme. Our experience suggests that areas of interest are often identified during a programme as participants consider case studies, and then linking to a previously unidentified theme becomes necessary.

The course requires the minimum of equipment and can be held almost anywhere. But we recommend finding out in advance as much as possible about the participants (see checklist below).

Getting Ready: A Checklist for Tutors

The Participants

- How many are expected?
- How many men? How many women?
- Are any of them taking early retirement or facing redundancy?
- Is the group multi-racial? Or is it predominantly one ethnic group?
- Have their partners in retirement been invited, where appropriate?
- Is it known what the participants are expecting from the programme?

The Venue

- Does the room have easy access?
- Are the chairs both comfortable and easy to move? (The small group work will involve a fair amount of furniture re-arrangement.)
- Is there at least one table for the display of handouts, leaflets etc.?
- Is there a suitable surface (display boards, plain wall, cupboards etc.) on which to stick flipchart sheets?
- Are the catering facilities satisfactory? (Remember participants may welcome tea or coffee breaks during sessions.)

Basic Equipment

all sessions
Flipchart stand
Adequate supply of flipchart paper
Assortment of pens, preferably coloured
Means of displaying several sheets at a time (according to surface: pins, Blu-Tack, etc.)
Photocopies of handouts as necessary
Name Badges

Optional extras
TV set, video recorder
OHP (if using handouts as transparencies)
Tape recorder (final session, and to pre-record scripts of
videos if desired)

Preparation and Evaluation

We think tutors would find it helpful to evaluate or assess
their own experiences of the programme in a systematic way.

- How well did each activity go? Which part did not work
  well?
- Did the participants respond well to the learning/teaching
  methods suggested? If not, were you able to select an
  alternative method?
- How effectively did you draw on participants' own
  experiences?
- How effectively did you help participants explore the steps
  of the Coping with Change model?
- Was the handout material satisfactory? Would you change
  it on another occasion?

We are aware that running a course of this kind places great
demands on the tutor, not least on his or her self-confidence
in facing a group without the support of a pre-arranged
programme and a panel of 'experts'. However, we can only
say that we have found the effort worthwhile and we hope
others will be encouraged to experiment. The Coping with
Change model provides a framework for a pre-retirement
programme which will meet participants' individual needs
and help them to make what is often a difficult period of
transition a time of personal growth and development.

Part Two: The Coping with Change Model in Action

The Meaning of Retirement

Stages and method

1. Getting started (introductions, includes icebreaker)
2. Getting to know you (additional icebreaker)
3. What does retirement mean to you? (buzz groups with or without trigger video, small group work followed by report back)
4. Social and economic context (tutor's presentation followed by general discussion)

Purpose

This material is intended to be used in the first session, setting the scene for the remainder of the programme. The aim is to create a relaxed yet purposeful atmosphere which participants will find supportive and which will be conducive to learning. Participants begin to get to know each other (Stages 1 and 2), and are then encouraged to articulate their thoughts about retirement and explore their own feelings, both positive and negative (Stage 3). The tutor can then widen the context by engaging participants in a discussion about retirement as a social construct and about society's changing attitudes to older people (Stage 4).

Options

The outline suggested here may be adapted to suit a variety of circumstances. For instance, if participants come from the same organisation, they may know each other already so elaborate introductions will be unnecessary. However, the nature of the course and domestic arrangements will still need to be explained. With a two-day course it is preferable to organise a preliminary meeting a week or two before the event when this material may be used (see page 21). If time is limited, consider circulating some of the background information beforehand in written form, putting the question 'What does retirement mean to you?' in an introductory letter, and preparing a summary of replies for the first meeting.

Information for tutors

Background notes about the social and economic context of retirement which could be used as a basis for the presentation in Stage 4 are on pages 30–32.

Practical points

Advice about seating arrangements and its implications is on page 32. Suggestions about names and name badges are on page 33. Notes on the optional use of videos are on page 34.

Resources used in Stages 1-4

Labels or lapel badges
Flipchart, flipchart paper, pens, Blu-Tack
Optional: television set, video recorder, CHRE video 'Focus on Health, Focus on Retirement' (and see note on page 76).

Course material

Learning activities begin on page 34.

| Information for Tutors: | *The Social and Economic Context of Retirement* |

The idea of preparing for retirement is a fairly recent one. And so too is the concept of a fixed age at which employment should cease. At the turn of this century, there were no state pensions. Most people who were too old to earn a living had to rely on charity and the Poor Law, though occupational pensions for some civil servants had been introduced as early as 1859. The Old Age Pension Act of 1908 introduced a small non-contributory means-tested pension for applicants over the age of 70. Better provision was made by the Widows, Orphans and Old Age Contributory Pensions Act of 1925. It was not until 1942 that the Beveridge Report (which established the foundations of the modern Welfare State) introduced the idea of basic rate pensions on retirement from work for men from 65 and for women from 60. However, in 1942 there was no idea of making retirement compulsory.

Since 1960 the idea of relating the amount of pension to previous earnings has grown. In 1961 graduated pensions were introduced, and from 1975 pensions became earnings related (a practice which is now being phased out). Meanwhile, over the years a number of employers have introduced their own pension schemes (either contributory, non-contributory or shared between employer and employee) until in the 1980s even small employers have instituted schemes through regular contributions to insurance companies. Now government legislation is proposing a shift away from reliance on the state pension towards the development of personal, portable pensions built up over a number of years by the individual when in paid employment.

Demographic Trends

In this century the number of people actually reaching retirement age has increased dramatically. Expectation of life at birth has risen from 48.5 years for men and 52.4 years for women in 1901 to 71.8 and 77.7 years respectively in 1985. Life expectancy at age 60 is now 16.6 more years for men and 21 years for women. Consequently there has been a steady increase in the proportion of the population over retirement age: 9.3 per cent in 1921 compared to 19 per cent in 1988.

So the second half of this century has seen a new development human experience. Most people can expect to spend some years in relative leisure after the end of their working lives, with at least a basic pension as of right. Many men and women will have 20 or more years of retirement with an occupational pension which protects to some extent the standard of living they enjoyed while at work.

Changing Patterns of Work

Since the Second World War Britain has changed from a society whose economy depended on heavy industry to an electronic and computer-based one. With this change came 'early retirement', redundancy and recession, and long-term unemployment. But because of the steady fall in the birth rate in the late 1960s and 1970s, the last ten years of this century may well see again a shortage of workers of all ages under 60, and bring into question the need for a fixed retirement age. Government encouragement to employers to train and re-train staff is countered by pleas from the voluntary sector, in particular, to offer relevant support – including information, counselling and guidance – for those who are still facing the problems of early retirement and redundancy.

Married women make up an increasing proportion of the workforce. At the beginning of the century about 10 per cent of married women worked outside the home. Today nearly two-thirds are at work, a proportion which is still rising. However, women are often found in part-time low-paid jobs that do not qualify for occupational pensions. Retirement has been seen, typically, as an event in a man's life course. Most males are at school through childhood and adolescence; go to work in late adolescence or early adulthood; continue to work through marriage and parenthood; retire from work in their early 60s. Pensions and benefits have often been seen only in this context. But it is now being recognised that women experience retirement differently – as part of a life course which may contain a period of withdrawal from work to look after young children, a return to part-time employment without benefits, and a further withdrawal from work to care for elderly parents.

Even less attention has so far been paid to the experience of retirement in minority cultures.

More emphasis is being placed on the ability of individuals in mid-life to cope with unprecedented social change. Yet these people, especially those now in their 50s, are men who grew up with the expectation of full-time work from school-leaving age to statutory retirement age and women who were accustomed to regard themselves as dependants – expectations which were reflected in the form and content of their initial education.

Attitudes to Age

One side-effect of a fixed retirement age has been the tendency to discriminate against people in mid-life in obtaining paid employment. Some employers seem to consider that anyone over the age of 40 is 'too old to learn new skills' or 'not able to work as fast as younger people'. This tends to influence the way people think about their own abilities, and some come to believe this discrimination is 'true'. Western civilisation has gone through a phase of being prejudiced in favour of youth and against age, and also of valuing contribution to society only in terms of paid employment. 'Useful and youthful' contrasts sharply with 'useless and old'. Images of older people and the ageing process in the media are often derogatory or mocking.

Yet the evidence is that ageing does not necessarily mean illness. Many older people are healthy, and many people in mid-life have found that it is possible to arrest or slow down what was taken to be inevitable decline by adopting a more healthy lifestyle.

Practical Points

1. Seating arrangements for small groups

There are a number of ways in which seats can be arranged in order to make discussion easier and the whole occasion more enjoyable. Much depends on the space available, the purpose of the event and the relative ease or difficulty in arranging the furniture. Experience shows that most adults prefer less formal seating arrangements, especially if the furniture enables them (with the tutor) to adapt and change the format to suit the learning session taking place.

Formal (with a table)

- reminiscent of a board meeting where formal business or negotiation takes place
- each member has an allocated space which can help them to feel safe and assist less mobile people with getting up and down
- the leader is in a prominent position but cannot necessarily be seen easily by all the members
- useful if papers are to be circulated and referred to, for writing purposes, or just resting or leaning one's elbows or hands.

Slightly less formal (with table)

- similar to the more formal arrangement with the rectangular table but the leader is less prominent and all the members can see each other
- inhibiting if visual or aural aids are to be used during the session

Less formal (without table)

- a natural seating arrangement reminiscent of a family group at home
- chairs easily moved if visual aids are to be used during the session
- leader not in prominent position
- difficult if members wish or need to write or refer to any papers.

Formal (without table)

- leader in the most prominent position reminiscent of a choir or orchestra in session, and can be seen by all group members
- slightly more flexibility in the amount of space available for each member, depending on the type and size of chair
- very convenient arrangement if visual or aural aids are to be used
- difficult for writing (unless chairs have swing writing top attachments) or for resting elbows and hands
- difficult to escape the attentive eye of the leader or make non-verbal signs to any other member
- easily changed into other arrangements if necessary during the session.

If there is a choice of chairs consider their ease of movement, the space available and the shape of the group seating.

Easy chairs induce sleep and make writing difficult. Conference chairs are usually comfortable, easy to move and suitable for reading and writing.

Remember to include at least two extra upright chairs in any group for back sufferers and allow space for a wheelchair if you have a disabled member.

When people arrive they will be conscious of the existing seating arrangements. For example, a large circle of empty chairs may be a neat arrangement but very off-putting. Why not leave the chairs scattered around informally, then invite the group to turn their chairs towards you (this gives you a choice of where to stand) when you start.

2. Names

Two things should be borne in mind:

1. People differ in what they like to be called, and this should be respected. There is no need to force anyone to be more or less familiar than he or she wishes to be.
2. Name labels are useless if they are illegible. Failing eyesight is a common characteristic of later life, therefore labels should be on the large side. You can give the lead by writing your own name in large letters with thick fibre-tipped pen in advance and inviting others to follow your

example. When discussion takes place in a room with tables, desk labels are better than lapel badges.

3. Optional use of video in Stage 3

If you decide to use the CHRE video 'What Does Retirement Mean to You?' in Stage 3, state your reasons, show the whole video, identify the issues brought out, together with those raised by the members, eg the video includes 'loss of identity', 'changes in finance', 'importance of planning', 'women cope better than men'. There is more information about using videos on pages 76 and 79.

Course Material

Stage 1. Getting started

Spend a few minutes (no more than ten) introducing yourself to the group and setting out the main purpose of the event. If you have prepared a printed programme in advance, describe the general outline and some of the ways in which you propose the group should work together. Remember to mention the domestic arrangements such as lunch, tea/coffee breaks, finishing times, cloakroom facilities, car parking or public transport arrangements. Invite questions on any points, also any comments, particularly on the course outline or general arrangements.

Activity

Begin the first activity by inviting participants to sit in pairs (or simply speak to the person sitting next to them). Ask them to introduce themselves (name, where they come from), then share one nice thing that has happened to them during the last week. After five minutes ask each person to introduce his or her partner to the whole group.
This whole activity should take 20–30 minutes, depending on the size of the group.

Notes

This may be the first occasion on which some of the participants have been invited to begin a conversation with a 'stranger'; therefore the time you spend introducing this activity will be invaluable.

Try to observe the reactions of the participants. You may decide that they need more than the five minutes suggested. You may also sense that they are not ready to talk openly to the whole group in introducing their partners. If so, move straight into Stage 2 and delay the introduction of partners until the end of this second 'icebreaker'.

Stage 2. Getting to know you

Activity

Move into the second activity by inviting the participants to stand up and introduce themselves initially to one other person (preferably someone they haven't met before or seen for a long time). Suggest they do this by shaking hands and exchanging some general information (as in the first part of the previous activity) about themselves. After two or three minutes call 'Change'. Participants then find a different partner and repeat the process. Continue until everyone within the group has met informally. *This activity will take 15–20 minutes.*

Notes

As one of the main aims of this activity is to enable everyone to say 'hello' informally, it is important to observe how the introductions are progressing. Timing is crucial. If some people appear to be having difficulty in starting or maintaining conversations, call 'Change' earlier than planned. This activity can be energising, thereby enabling all participants to talk or listen as much or as little as they wish, while creating a friendly and relaxed atmosphere.

If you had opted to leave the 'introduction of partners' from Stage 1 until now, invite participants to 'seek out the person you first met and sit next to him or her, so that you can prompt each other if necessary'. Such a comment from the tutor encourages the group to feel that the exercise is really designed for their benefit and that they are not being placed under any pressure.

Stage 3. What does retirement mean to you?

It is useful to have written this question on a flipchart sheet in advance, and reveal it at this stage.

If you have some prior knowledge of the age of the participants, use this as a basis for your introduction to this activity. For example: 'Although many people here will not receive their state pension for some time, I'm sure we all have some thoughts about our own retirement – when it arrives. Many of us live with people in widely different age groups. What are their thoughts about their own retirement, or what do they think of ours? Have we ever asked them or discussed it with them? For those of us in the group who have partners, I wonder what they may be thinking about our retirement.'

By the judicious use of advance information, followed by questions such as these, you demonstrate to the group that you are inviting them personally to think about their own retirement – what it means to them. It is also probably the first time the word retirement has been used with the group, and the participants will be realising that you have set out your objectives for the course, and they are beginning to respond and work with you. In introducing the activity explain your reasons for inviting the participants to work in small groups. An important reason is that you want to begin recording as many of their comments as possible, and one of the easiest and most efficient ways to achieve this is to distribute flipchart sheets to each group.

Activity

Invite participants to work in groups of about four, and ask each group to consider the question 'What does retirement mean to you?' Suggest that each group nominates a writer and a rapporteur (could be the same person) to record the responses and speak about the group's comments in plenary session.
Allow 10 minutes for this.

Next ask the groups to identify the positive and negative statements they have made about their retirement by adding a plus or a minus in a coloured marker pen against each statement.
This should take about 5 minutes.

Bring the small groups together in plenary session, invite the rapporteur from each group in turn to display and 'talk to' the comments on the flipcharts. Encourage additional comments on any of the summaries, and display all flipchart sheets around the room, using wall space if possible.
This last phase will probably average 3 minutes for each presentation.

Notes

While this activity is proceeding, prepare the space for the flipcharts or move any visual aids you will be using in the next stage into position. Demonstrate to the group that you also have a task to do! Avoid sitting in the front in isolation, which could easily remind the group of their school-days and suggest that they are currently engaged in a 'supervised' exercise. In some instances you may feel like joining one or more of the groups for a few minutes to listen to (rather than guide) their discussions.

Be aware of the amount of time taken up with this activity. If it drifts too much out of your control the group may feel you haven't carried out your role efficiently. If your prepared timetable is disrupted because of the size of the group or the need to break into small groups, reduce the amount of time for discussion, explaining your actions, if necessary, to the group.

Options: There are two other approaches to this activity which have been used successfully. The first is to use the CHRE's trigger video as an aid to discussion. Play the video and follow the same procedure as in the previous method, but on this occasion preface the group discussions with the task 'Choose a statement on the video you most agree with, and one you disagree with'. By using this approach, many people who are reluctant to begin talking about their own retirement feel more able to comment on what someone else has said.

The second alternative is to substitute the questions 'What are you most looking forward to in your retirement?' and 'What are you least looking forward to?' Follow the same procedures, using small group discussions and feedback. Although these questions may seem to be more direct or even personal than the other, experience shows that they can generate intense discussion. If you decide to adopt this alternative, be aware of one or more people who may dominate the small group discussions with their own particular expectations or prejudices about their retirement.

Stage 4. Social and economic context of retirement

The work of the groups, now summarised on a number of displayed flipchart sheets, provides the opportunity to make a presentation in which retirement in the 1990s can be compared with retirement at the beginning of this century and its history traced in a social/economic context. The main purpose of this presentation is to enable the group to see themselves belonging to an age group who have experienced changes in their own and society's understanding of retirement. It also encourages reflection and further analysis of the positive and negative aspects of retirement which emerged in the discussion in Stage 3.

Prevailing attitudes towards ageing can be compared with those of 25 or 50 years ago and people's perception of being or becoming old can be considered in the context of health or of pensions and paid work.

Activity

Begin by asking the group what the response would be if their grandparents or even great grandparents had considered the question 'What does retirement mean to you?' Encourage feedback and reminiscence, especially if some people in the group can actually remember their great grandparents.

Lead on to a brief summary of the history and social context of retirement (see Information for Tutors). Emphasise key factors such as the emergence and development of occupational and state pensions; give particular emphasis to the historical approach to retirement as something which only concerned men. Be aware that for some people in the group the British social history of retirement may have little meaning and encourage cross-cultural references. Also encourage the group to discuss the implications of legislative and social changes concerning retirement during this century.

Sum up by going over again the inevitable movement from the structure of paid work to the relative freedom of retirement. Explore ways in which the experience of those retiring from paid work can be seen to be both similar to and different from the

experience of those now engaged in unpaid work. Note the objectives of the pre-retirement course or programme in this context and stress the value of setting aside time to think through some of the issues, hopes, aspirations, fears or apprehensions associated with retirement.
This could take about 30 minutes.

Notes

This is the first presentation to the group and it is important to outline the purposes of the course and involve the group as much as possible. Setting out the historical factors and social and economic context of retirement will encourage people to talk and/or reminisce quite readily, and it is important to allow them this time.

Be prepared for the fact that recent changes in legislation in, for example, personal taxation can raise some important issues. If questions of this kind are raised by the group at this point, either pause and discuss them immediately (if it is a matter of information not opinion) or list the questions on a flipchart and undertake to return to them later in the course.

Looking at Life Changes

Stages and method

5. Understanding change (explanatory talk followed by small group work)
6. The process of transition (tutor-led discussion)
7. Letting go and looking ahead (small group work followed by general discussion)

Purpose

This material provides participants with information on change and transition, and enables them to consider the nature of change and the way this influences their perception of retirement. Participants are encouraged to explore the variety of changes they have experienced in their lives (Stage 5) and are introduced to the idea of 'coping with change' (Stage 6); the tutor then discusses the importance of 'letting go' and its relevance to retirement (Stage 7).

Options

Time allowed: in preparing the outline of the course it is important to allow sufficient time for these three stages and the two which follow. There is a temptation to move forward too quickly towards problem-solving and information exchange, but unless participants thoroughly understand the central proposition that retirement is part of a sequence of life changes, and the way in which transition is experienced, the purpose of the rest of the resource materials will be lost. In a two-day course half- to a whole day may be spent on Stages 1–9. In a course of six or eight sessions that extends over several weeks two sessions may be spent on these stages (see pages 21–23).

Information for tutors

Background notes about change and transition that could form the basis for the explanatory talk in Stage 5 are on page 41, together with some suggestions for further reading.

Practical points

Some hints about using discussion are on page 42.

Resources used in Stages 5-7

Flipchart, flipchart paper, pens, Blu-Tack
Notepaper, pencils
Handout 1: Transition curve; and Handout 2: Coping with Change model

Course material

Learning activities begin on page 44.
Handouts 1 and 2 are on pages 103–104.

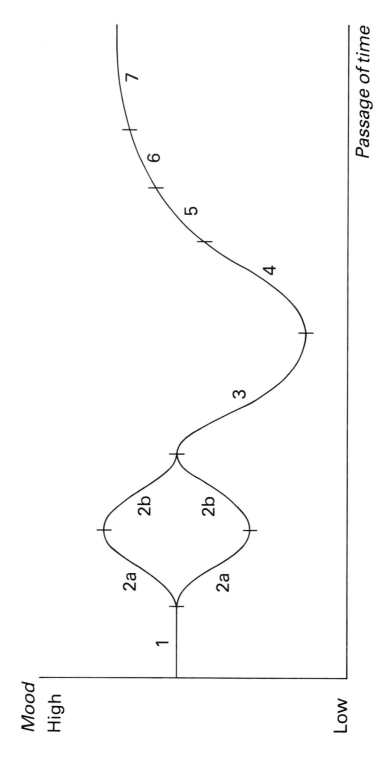

Figure 7 *Seven-phase model of transition (reproduced with permission from* Life-span Development, *L Sugarman, Methuen, 1986, attributed to Hopson, 1981*).*

* Hopson, B in *Counseling Psychologist* Vol 9(2) 1981.

Information for Tutors:

About Change and Transition

The experience of change is an inevitable consequence of living. Some changes are anticipated (or predictable), such as growing from a child into an adolescent, and from an adolescent into an adult. Some changes are not anticipated (or non-predictable), such as being involved in a car crash or winning the football pools. Changes – whether they can be predicted or not – may be warmly welcomed at one extreme (getting married, perhaps) or deeply resented at the other (being made redundant, perhaps).

For any major change in life to be accepted, an element of time must be involved, which psychologists call 'the period of transition'. Undergoing and subsequently recalling these 'life events' enables people to build up their own special knowledge and understanding of such times. Hopson and Adams (1976) describe the period of transition as 'a discontinuity in a person's life-space'. Not everyone will experience the same transitional event in the same way. People's experiences of retirement will vary enormously. But in any period of transition it is likely that people will be aware that there *is* discontinuity in their life, and that new 'behavioural responses' will be needed to meet it. Whether the change in the life course is intentional, a sudden surprise, or a growing awareness of decreasing stability, it will trigger a cycle of reactions and feelings that is predictable enough to be mapped.

Each stage is associated with particular feelings. To paraphrase Sugarman's text:

1. *Shock* – the feeling of being overwhelmed, and in shock. Not knowing what to do.
2. *Denial* – the desire to reduce the problem by trivialisation, possible denial and feelings of euphoria.
3. *Depression or self-doubt* – as awareness increases, conflicts between needs and feelings arise. These are suppressed, resulting in depression.
4. *Acceptance of reality* – 'letting go'. Up to this point the individual has 'held on' to the past; at this stage the chance to 'let go and look ahead' begins. Feelings are expressed and are more optimistic.
5. *Testing* – a period of experimentation occurs in which new roles, behaviours and life-styles are tested and 'tried on for size'.

6. *Searching for meaning* – in this phase the individual thinks through the feelings and changes that have just taken place, and attempts to gain an understanding of what has happened and why.
7. *Acceptance* – at this stage a new life-style (role, behaviours, attitudes) becomes integrated within the individual's existing concepts and beliefs and the process of transition is completed. On the transition graph, higher self-esteem after the transition denotes personal development of some kind.

The model is, of course, more representative than specific. The cycle of reactions is as applicable for the happy and welcomed changes in life as for the sad, unwelcomed ones. Some people have clear recollections, both of the stages and their feelings of a transition, while others do not. The feelings they recall may be of elation and happiness and it is only on further thought that they remember moments of apprehension or searching. Others appear to become stuck in a particular stage of transition (and acknowledge it), while others may almost seem not to have experienced it at all.

Suggestions for further reading

Davis, F., *Yearning for Yesterday*, New York: Free Press, 1979.
Erikson, E.H., *Identity and the Life Cycle*, New York: Norton, 1980.
George, L., *Role Transitions in Later Life*, Belmont: Wadsworth, 1980.
Hopson, B. and Adams J. in J. Hayes and B. Hopson (eds), *Transition: Understanding and Managing Personal Change*, London: Martin Robertson, 1976.
Sheehy, G., *Passages: Predictable Crises of Adult Life*, New York: Dutton, 1976.

Practical Points:

Using Discussion

Hints for discussion group leaders

- Taking part in a group discussion will be a novel experience for some people and they will need time to adjust.
- If possible use a gentle tone of voice – it is far more effective.
- Encourage the group to avoid generalisations, and to make

statements in the first person: 'I think this . . .' rather than 'people ought to think . . .'

- On the other hand, help the group to understand the general significance of the personal stories that different people tell.
- Avoid the use of jargon or others in the group may copy you.
- Be conscious that there are sequences of growth and development in any discussion.
- Be aware of the quiet or shy members. Their silence may not indicate their lack of participation. They may be waiting to be brought into the discussion. Encourage the hesitant by asking for opinions (not information); eg 'What about you, Basil, how do you feel about it?'
- Be aware of the difficult group members. Tactfully restrain the over-enthusiastic; eg 'Can we stop you there for just a moment, Joan, and ask the others how they feel about it?' It may be tempting to 'put them down', compete with them, ignore them or demonstrate frustration or annoyance with their behaviour. It is much more constructive to interrupt them when they make a particularly valid point relating to the main theme. Build on or analyse that point immediately and draw on the other group members. Remember that the judicial use of buzz groups can be an effective technique in focusing on one particular task in order to allow the group to return to the main theme.
- Be prepared to release the leadership role temporarily and allow it to pass to another. It will be counter-productive if a member who sought out information or advice for the group (with its prior agreement) is not allowed time to report back.
- Be prepared to answer a direct question on a point of fact or information. If you do not know, say so openly and invite others to give the answer.
- Be ready to try a new or different approach or style of leadership and explain why you are doing it. Resist the temptation to give a series of mini-lectures in response to questions from the group which may not have a simple answer.
- Be prepared to bring together all the main points at the end of the discussion, adding extra factual information then, if necessary.

How to conduct a discussion

1. *Brief opening remarks* – eg 'I suggest we start by looking at . . .' Probably only one or two people react. Ask 'What is your opinion?'
2. *To increase involvement* – say 'Shall we consider those first responses in more detail?' *or* 'What do others think about

that statement . . . ?' More members participate. Check how many join in and encourage (if necessary) any member who is obviously anxious to establish a position in the debate.

3. *Keeping it going* – check how much time has been spent on the task or issue. If necessary share your concern about timing with the participants. They will appreciate your concern and decide with you on strict time-keeping or agree on a degree of flexibility.

4. *To encourage conclusions* – say 'We have had a wide range of opinions on . . . Are we now ready to come to some conclusions?' If discussion has been full and frank there will be a positive reaction to your question. If not it *could* mean that the discussion has not proceeded at a pace which matches the group's abilities.

5. *To conclude the discussion* – say 'We now have just eight minutes left. I would like to summarise the conclusions we have reached in our discussions and indicate those issues which we still feel are unsolved or on which there are strong minority opinions.' The members feel that they have achieved something and that you have kindly yet firmly kept the discussion within the given terms of reference.

Course Material

Stage 5. Understanding change

The realisation that retirement as a period or phase in life can be seen as a social construct, and that experiences of retirement differ not only in generational but also individual ways, forms the basis for the consideration of the number and nature of many changes in life. Some of these changes, such as becoming an adult, are familiar to all; others, such as being involved in an accident, may be familiar only to one or two members of the group.

Activity

Begin by giving a brief explanatory talk on the purpose of this activity, by which participants are encouraged to consider 'coping with change' as an important way of looking at a variety of experiences through which they have lived.
Allow 10 minutes for this.

Divide the participants into groups of four. Ask each group to draw ten columns on the flipchart paper, representing the decades in a person's age from 1–100 years (ie 1–10 years, 11–20 years, 21–30 years and so on). In each column list the events (changes) which a person of 60 years of age will probably have experienced in his or her life-time (eg starting school, starting a job, starting/finishing a relationship). Next, place the letter (1) against those events which were predictable and (2) against those which were unpredictable. *After 15 minutes ask the groups to display their completed sheets so that the whole group can see the similarities, differences and possible omissions.*

Now hand out the paper and pencils and ask participants, working on their own, to identify one predictable and one unpredictable event in their lives and see if they can remember the length of time it took to live through the whole period of change. *Allow 10 minutes for this.*

Now ask for some reactions. For example, 'Were any of you surprised at the length of time it took to cope with some changes in life?' Go on to distribute Handouts 1 and 2 and show how the activity the group has just completed relates to the model. Demonstrate to the group that retirement, as an *event*, may be predictable and welcomed by some and yet unwelcomed by others. This implies no criticism, but simply acknowledges the differences between people. Refer back to the psychological theory and also to the experiences of the group doing the exercises, and summarise this stage as illustrating, and accepting, that retirement is one of the major changes in life, and that preparing for retirement is, in effect, preparing to cope with change. *Allow a total of 45 minutes for the whole activity.*

Notes

It is important that participants understand right from the beginning the purposes of being engaged in this activity. The basis for the whole programme is the understanding of the nature of life changes and the experience of transition in which all participants can subscribe to the learning process. In practice, the time spent on this stage could vary considerably according to the schedule, the composition of the group and their motivation to learn. It is important to use as many, or as few, examples of predictable and non-predictable events as necessary to match the level of the group learning. An opportunity may occur to ask additional questions such as 'Think of a predictable change in your lives which you have experienced, such as leaving school. Did you approach that change willingly or reluctantly? Can you recall? (For example, some people know that at the date they left school, they were reluctant to leave.) During this experience, do you recall talking to anyone in particular about your reluctance? Did he or she make it easier? How did you eventually adjust? Looking back, what have you learnt from that experience which, had you known then, would have helped you to adjust more easily? Such questions enable participants to begin thinking about their own abilities to cope.

If time allows, you may wish to consider anticipating a later stage by asking the participants to think of other changes in life people will probably experience after 60 years of age. Note that some participants will probably identify illness, bereavement and loneliness, and others may suggest moving house or returning to an earlier home. These ideas will be picked up again in Stage 8.

Stage 6. The process of transition

In moving on to this stage, you will need to explain that the period of transition represents a period of time, and in this context the period of time lived through in experiencing, adjusting to and accepting a change in life. Point out that many changes happen gradually (such as relating age to perceptions of health) and may be less noticeable than other more abrupt changes. Also emphasise the potential for growth or development or opportunity which are inherent in many changes.

Activity

After your introduction, ask the whole group to consider an unexpected (non-predictable) event (change). Say, for instance, 'You open your post and find you have won the Holiday of Your Dreams in a competition. How do you feel? What are your first reactions?' List comments on a flipchart as they are offered. Then obtain a list of 'Your second or more considered thoughts after some time has passed'. On a flipchart place 'A' as the starting point of the happy event and interpret the first and subsequent thoughts about the change as a line graph between the starting point 'A' and finishing point 'B'. Demonstrate that the life-satisfaction level at point 'A' probably showed an increase at point 'B'.

Repeat the exercise by asking the participants to recall a 'less happy' event in their lives. Say 'Do not reveal this event, but try to recall your feelings when it happened'. List first and subsequent feelings/reactions as in the previous example, and demonstrate that, at the end of the transition period, the life-satisfaction level has probably lowered.

Both examples demonstrate that the feelings and steps throughout the period of transition are normal reactions and some of them (eg loss) are common to all changes in life. Refer to the transition curve (Handout 1) to show how normal reactions form a predictable pattern.
Allow 35 minutes for this activity.

Notes

It is particularly important to emphasise that, while a predictable pattern of stages in any transitional period can be ascertained, the sequence of or the amount of time in (or even the awareness of) these stages can vary because of many factors, including the nature of the change and the experience of the individual in coping with similar changes in the past.

Therefore the transition period into 'retirement' should not be seen simply as a 'problem' time. The stages many people may have reached in, for example, adjusting to the idea of a revised income or a different use of time could be reflected as positive feelings on their life-satisfaction graph, whereas for others the intense concern about one particular aspect of expected change (such as missing the friendship of colleagues and being alone) is a real stumbling block to coping/managing the process of transition. The recognition of such differences between people and the opportunity to consider a progressive and meaningful approach to control, manage and live through these experiences successfully, demonstrate the value of regular reference to the steps suggested in the Coping with Change model.

Stage 7. Letting go and looking ahead

In Stage 6 the participants considered their own feelings in practical examples of two changes which may occur in life. In this stage they are invited to think of one, sometimes lingering, feature of a transition experience – 'letting go'.

It is worth giving a few indicators or triggers to enable the following small group discussions to be fruitful before setting the tasks. The 'letting go' of an old or familiar situation often appears to be negative, but the action or process can be very positive indeed. For example, a happy event like a job promotion may require leaving many friends, but the actual 'letting go' does not necessarily require losing friendship, but rather accepting, perhaps, that the frequency of meetings, the habits which have been formed in association together, must end.

Activity

Ask the participants to meet in the same groups of four to discuss the questions 'What is involved in letting go?', 'Is letting go always a difficult process?', 'Can you think of any phase or change in life where you impeded the new beginning by refusing or delaying the "ending"? Use only examples you are perfectly willing to share with the group.' Explain that there will be no formal report-back session, but that you will conduct an open discussion for 15 minutes at the end.
Allow 15 minutes for this.

Bring the whole group together again and engage in open discussion of the same questions debated in the small groups. Sum up this stage with the recognition that the experience of a period of transition is an inevitable consequence of change, and that we can sometimes impede or accelerate the process by the way we let go of the previous phase.
Allow 15 minutes for this.

Notes

This exercise is the culmination of the series designed to enable participants to analyse the meaning of retirement for them, to draw on their experiences of coping with change in their lives, and demonstrate that the whole basis of any course or programme of preparation for retirement is the knowledge, skills and attitude relating to life changes and transitions. Many of the questions which the participants have addressed are of a reflective nature. They are designed to encourage participants to focus on particular issues without necessarily sharing their thoughts openly with other members. They are also designed to demonstrate the steps or stages in the Coping with Change model, and it is important to allow as much time as possible at each stage. For example, to consider 'what to do in retirement' before exploring experiences of transition in a variety of life events, and before taking stock, denies the individual a sound foundation on which to design a plan, consider options, seek sources of relevant information and relate to those with whom he or she may live or maintain close contact in this new phase in life.

Preparing for Change

Stages and method

8. Retirement and change (review to date, small group work with or without report back)
9. Identifying themes of change (tutor-led discussion)

Purpose

This material is intended to enable tutors and participants to use the remainder of the course time in the most appropriate way. Participants should feel that the ownership of the course is very much in their hands from now on. The tutor can now show in detail the relevance of the Coping with Change model to preparation for retirement. Participants look carefully at the changes which retirement will bring to their lives and consider whether these will be changes for the better or for the worse (Stage 8); tutors and participants together group issues into 'themes' (Stage 9), and decide which they will examine in detail and in what order.

Options

Stage 8 does in fact follow on directly from Stage 7 and may be taken as a continuation of the previous session, but it is presented here separately since it is important that enough time is allowed for review and forward planning. If these two stages are rushed through at the end of what is already quite a demanding theoretical exposition, participants may well be confused about the choices now open to them. Tutors operating this course single-handed will find they need some time after the competition of Stage 9 to reorganise the material for the remainder of the course, and perhaps also to give participants time to do some preparatory thinking about whatever the next theme is to be.

Information for tutors

More about developing themes and their relationship to the model can be found on page 50.

Practical points

Hints on how to handle this session are on page 53.

Resources used in Stages 8 and 9

Flipchart, flipchart paper, pens, Blu-Tack
Flipchart sheets compiled in earlier stages

Course material

Learning activities begin on page 55.

| Information for Tutors: | # About the Themes and their Relationship to the Model |

At this point in the course participants are invited to identify their main concerns about the changes retirement will bring. The following sections of resource material examine a range of issues grouped into four themes – time, finance, health and relationships. There is, of course, an apparent contradiction here, in that we appear to be predetermining an open choice programme, but we have found in practice with many groups that these themes almost always occur, though with varying degrees of emphasis. The only exceptions have been in groups where the participants have a particular occupation-related problem (with tied housing, for instance) which can usually be foreseen. Ways of incorporating issues of this kind are indicated in the text. *It is important that the themes are selected and used in the order identified by the participants.*

Groups do not always identify all these themes. For example, on some occasions participants have only identified money issues as being of interest to them in the first instance. But in developing the theme it becomes apparent that money issues raise questions about the use of time, about aspects of life-style, about other people and other places. As the programme proceeds, participants begin to identify further themes which can then be developed in turn.

Each theme is sub-divided into topics and each topic contains activities which are closely related to the Coping with Change model (see Figure 8). The development of the themes is inter-related. Activities in different themes have a similar function though they are related to a specific area of interest. For example, in the theme Relationships the activity in Topic A deals with identifying the effects of transition; in the theme Health this step of the model appears in Topic A.2. Figure 8 shows how the topics and activities of all the themes relate to the model.

The themes are also inter-related because issues can hardly ever be considered in isolation. Possible links from one theme to another are indicated in the Options paragraph under each theme.

Steps in the Coping with Change model	Theme – Time				Theme – Finance						Theme – Relationships						Theme – Health			
	Topic A	Topic B			Topic A	Topic B					Topic A	Topic B					Topic A	Topic B		
	1	1	2	3	1	1	2	3	4	5	1	1	2	3	4	5	1	1	2	3
Identifying effects of transition	■				■						■							■		
Taking stock – identifying – understanding key issues		■	■			■		■	■			■	■				■			
Considering choices/options				■			■	■	■				■	■	■	■			■	
Making choices				■					■				■	■	■					■
Taking action				■						■						■				■
Reassessment	*	*	*	*	*	*	*	*	*	*	*	*	*	*	*	*	*	*	*	*

Key ■ represents the step(s) of the Coping with Change model considered in that activity.
 * this stage of the model is undertaken by participants as they evaluate their decisions as time passes.

Figure 8   *The Themes and Their Relationships to the Coping with Change Model*

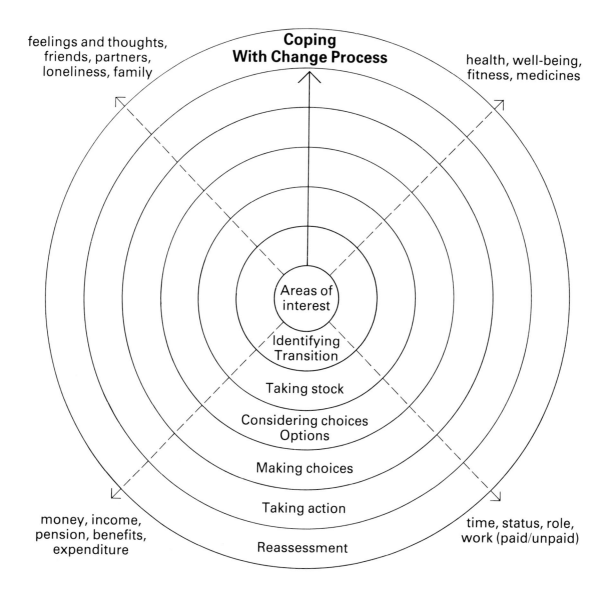

Figure 9   *Diagram of the Relationship between the Coping with Change Model and the Practical Themes*

Practical Points

How to handle this session

A note of caution must be sounded about the way the long lists compiled by the participants in their groups in Stage 8 are brought under the heading of major themes. Both from background reading and experience the tutor will realise that almost all the issues brought forward will eventually cluster under the themes of health, finance, relationships and time. If, in fact, one (or more) of these themes does not emerge from the groups' lists there is a strong temptation for the tutor to suggest it should be included.

We recommend that this temptation is resisted for the following reasons. If the whole programme proceeds along the route suggested in these materials, it will be evident that any one change at the time of retirement is closely intertwined with at least one other or even more. For example, if a group puts foward only two themes of change such as finance and time, during the exploration of these themes other factors, such as friendships or health issues around immobility or perceptions of ageing, may well emerge. This is why we have developed the use of the case study on the Wyldes family as one of our major teaching/learning resources. We suggest that it is used as a prototype and adapted according to local circumstances and the tutor's knowledge of the group.

It is therefore extremely important at Stage 9 to negotiate some flexibility with the group around the exploration of the themes. In this way you will avoid simply producing four or more 'set subjects' in a given allocation of time. Moreover, each theme links with the model, especially the 'task' or problem-solving step. Given the number of changes that the participants have identified, they will now be more able to consider where they are at present in, for example, the transition period of the theme of finance. Some may have already prepared to a large extent for their retirement, and be on the upward curve, past 'making choices' and into 'taking action'. Others may be at the preliminary stages of either shock or elation. Working together in a group is a recognition of the different stages and variety of experiences of the participants. The opportunity for the tutor to harness those experiences with the anxieties often present in the various steps of understanding should not be lost.

Practical experience has shown that team-teaching (with two or more tutors working together) during this stage of the programme in particular is very rewarding. For example, if one tutor writes on the flipchart while the other engages in the determining of the clusters of changes with the group, a real team spirit is engendered, and the tutor 'scribe' can also contribute and/or question the participants as part of the process.

If Stage 9 comes at the end of the programme for the first day, or if the group will not meet again for some time (even one week), it is important to provide a link with the next meeting. For example, distribute any appropriate handout materials and invite participants to consider the nature and extent of their own future contributions to the rest of the programme. Some may have relevant expertise they are willing to share, others may volunteer to do some research on a particular issue for the whole group and/or pursue one or more sources of information for themselves, while others may wish to reflect before taking any further action.

The following preparation may be needed for the themes.

Theme time

In Topic B.3 participants are invited to share materials relating to their interests and leisure activities with others. Participants will need advance warning.

Theme finance

It is helpful to participants if they are aware of their financial position in retirement (ie their state, occupational and personal pensions) before attending this programme. The letters of invitation sent to the participants could include the Budget Sheets (Handout 7) together with a reminder to make certain that they are aware of the approximate amounts of their future pensions. This information is readily available from their employer's Pensions Department and/or the insurance companies in the case of personal pensions and free-standing Additional Voluntary Contribution (AVC) schemes. If outside speakers are involved, it is important for the tutor to brief them in advance, giving the approximate, or range of, pensions and lump sums (if applicable) of the participants they will be meeting.

Theme health

It is important to know well in advance if any participants have a specific disability for which special preparation (for example, seating or dietary requirements) may be necessary. All the tutors need to be aware of these and of other less obvious factors such as deafness or poor sight.

Theme relationships

The approach suggested in the 'I feel . . . will you?' activity, though often used successfully with other age groups, may present difficulties with older people. The less experienced tutor should be very familiar with the material before using it with a pre-retirement group.

<table>
<tr><td>

Course Material

</td></tr>
</table>

Stage 8. Retirement and change

At this stage the participants are invited to review the progress they have made together in the programme so far, and to use that collective knowledge and experience to determine the nature and timing of the rest of the course.

Using this approach, the participants should more fully understand the meaning of, and accept, the shared ownership of the programme which the tutor demonstrated from the first letter of invitation.

The group's progress through the Coping with Change model can now be demonstrated by the tutor initiating discussion about each of the seven previous stages and emphasising the relevance of each stage by reference to the model. On the basis of this experience the group can then look carefully and critically at the changes which retirement will bring to their lives, and consider to what extent these will be changes for the better or for the worse.

Activity

Divide participants into groups of four. Say 'Make a list of the changes which you think everybody will experience at retirement. Use the flipchart sheets you completed when we were talking about "What does retirement mean to you?" as a guide if you wish' – (or the 60+ columns from Stage 5 if these were completed).
Allow 10 minutes for this.

On a separate sheet (or using different coloured pens) the groups could also identify those changes which may occur only to some people. Put all the summaries on display and invite participants to walk around (if possible) and discuss the lists informally.
Allow 15 minutes for this.

Notes

Share with the group your reasons for inviting them to do this exercise. From their point of view they have considered this question earlier in the programme, or before they arrived, and now they are being asked to go through the same process again.

But by considering what retirement means to them, what it may have meant to their parents or grandparents, how they are part of a particular, or special, group (cohort) who are alive today with the prospect of a considerable period in 'active' retirement, the tutor has deliberately focused attention (through a series of stages) on the individual – it will be interpreted by the course participant as 'on me'.

Research shows that for many people attending a pre-retirement course this recognition of themselves as unique individuals, as people who not only have a bank of resources and experiences in life to draw on but who are also encouraged to share (even decide) the content of their own retirement programme, is a unique learning experience.

Therefore, taking time to invite the group to think through those changes which actually will occur in retirement (ie the inevitable periods of transition) helps them to focus from the general to the particular. The introduction to this exercise, in which the tutor and group review the earlier stages and look at the relevance of the stage they have reached in the Coping with Change model, is probably one of the most important tasks the tutor has undertaken in the course. A period of time, even a pause for reflection, is crucial; when people begin to feel and take responsibility for their own learning agenda, conflicting areas of uncertainty and apprehension are frequently present yet not openly expressed. It has been estimated that people are usually only prepared to offer about 70 per cent of their personal feelings about the changes that will occur at retirement. The other 30 per cent stays in their own domain. It is important that the tutor respects this and is constantly aware of the dangers of stepping outside this limit by, for example, asking personal questions or, even worse, by directing a personal question to one of the participants.

The ten minutes or so which may be available at the end for participants to walk around and discuss the lists informally can be viewed not only as a time for endorsement or challenge of views held, but also simply (yet equally as important) as a time to 'stretch one's legs' after a lengthy period of sitting.

Stage 9. Identifying themes of change

At this stage participants will decide on the changes which they consider most important and which will form the content of the remaining programme. Here the tutor may also contribute as a group member so that the ensuing 'ownership' of the course may be seen as having been collectively and co-operatively developed. By bringing the total lists of changes together and grouping those with common features into 'themes', the participants will have recorded their own agendas around their retirement issues. For example, words like exercise, or diet, or mental activity naturally cluster under the familiar title or theme of health. This democratic process is then carried a stage further when collective decisions need to be taken on which themes will be examined in detail, and in what order, and in what amount of time – given each pre-retirement course has its own defined length.

Activity

From the display of flipchart sheets arising from the small discussion groups in Stage 8, begin *with the participants* to gather changes which are the same, or very similar, into clusters. Introduce the phrase 'major themes of change'. It is likely that the largest clusters will relate to issues about the use of time, about relationships, about finance and about health.

Next invite the participants to take a critical look at the 'components' of each cluster in turn. What are the key or critical points? Are any components missing?

Then ask the participants to vote on each major theme to place them in order of importance. Take time to confirm the order of importance established. Check that this is agreed by everybody and that some participants do not have concerns that their personal priority may be omitted.
Allow 45 minutes for the whole activity.

Notes

It is important to link the activities (which include tutor presentations and synthesis of quite complex theories) with the progressive steps in the Coping with Change model.

Within the time available, for the remainder of your programme, discuss the way the agreed themes can be treated and indicate to participants the ways they can prepare for and contribute to the remainder of their pre-retirement programme. Mention the links to the next session as appropriate (see Practical Points page 54). Tell the participants that all information collated on flipchart sheets during this meeting will remain on display throughout the rest of the course.

Themes of Change – Alternative Treatments: Time

Topics and method

A. Transition and time (tutor-led discussion)
B. Analysis and use of time
    B.1. Structure of Time (case study, discussion, two options)
    B.2. Analysis of work (small groups with leader, report back)
    B.3. Time management – what now? (prepared contributions plus goal-setting activity)

Purpose

This theme provides a structure by which participants are encouraged to consider changing patterns in their use of time and the extent to which the changes created by retirement can become opportunities for personal choice. First, participants review their experience of change in relation to the use of time (Topic A) and then they analyse the extent to which they control how they use their time at present (Topic B). Activities B.1–3 enable participants to take stock, consider their options, make choices and look towards future action. B.1 looks at the use of time in two case studies. B.2 continues the 'gains and losses' analysis, examining the meaning of work and what pursuits may have been prevented by the need to work. B.3 invites participants to share their current interests and determine future goals.

Options

The topics and activities are sequenced and take participants through most of the steps of the Coping with Change model. If other themes have been taken before this one, be aware of how links can be made to matters raised in other sessions. For instance: relationships – how partners may need to plan to spend some time together and some time separately (most activities in this theme will cross-refer quite naturally to relationships, in particular activities B.1 and B.2); health – how time should perhaps be set aside for exercise; money – how much time if any to allocate to part-time work. If moving house was an issue raised, build in some discussion about the extent to which location might affect the way in

Information for tutors

Sources for reference are on page 59.

Practical points

Hints on how to use a case study are on page 60.

Resources used in this theme

Flipchart, flipchart paper, pens
Notepaper and pencils
Handouts 3a and 3b: The Wyldes case study; 4a–d: Timetables, before and after retirement; 5: Analysis of work

Course material

Learning activities begin on page 62.
Handouts 3, 4 and 5 are on pages 105–111.

which time can be spent. If the structure of the course allows, invite participants beforehand to bring in information about local activities – societies, classes, clubs, and so on, in which they are interested – or about travel possibilities.

<table>
<tr><td>

Information for Tutors:

</td><td>

Sources for Reference

</td></tr>
</table>

The course materials which follow are intended to help participants to formulate a positive way of thinking about anticipated changes in the use of time. In working through the steps of the model – in taking stock, identifying issues, in moving on to making choices – the process described helps participants to become aware of the information they will need in planning future action. The experienced tutor will build up a file of local contacts and resources. The following titles indicate a starting point for reference for both tutor and participants.

Taking Stock: Being Fifty in the Eighties, by Charles Handy (BBC Publications, 1983).
The Time of Your Life (Help the Aged with the Health Education Council, first published 1979, many editions).

What Next – Focus on Health (CHRE, 1987) contains a number of worksheets, including a checklist that could be used in Activity B.2 (see page 64).

Decisions, Decisions! A Practical Guide to Problem Solving and Decision Making, by A. Leigh (IPM, 1983).

Organisations to contact:
University of the Third Age (write to U3A-National Office, 1 Stockwell Green, London SW9 9JF for the address of your nearest group).
Pre-Retirement Association, Nodus Building, University of Surrey, Guildford, Surrey for information about publications and local associations.
Volunteer Bureau or Council of Voluntary Service – under 'V' in your telephone directory.
REACH, 89 Southwark Street, London SE1 0HD.

Practical Points

When to use a case study

- When its use fits into the overall course objectives and that particular part of the course.
- When the members of the group are fairly well acquainted with each other.
- When you know the group has some knowledge of the issues involved.
- When you feel that this aid to learning will be more effective than any other for the issues being considered.
- When you know that the circumstances created in the study can enable members to identify with issues which concern them.
- When the group wishes to explore their attitudes and feelings without talking directly about themselves.

How to design a written case study

If you prefer to prepare your own case study, decide on the aims and objectives before writing the script. Accept the fact that the preparation will take time but can be an enjoyable exercise with rewarding results.

Some points to consider

What is the main purpose of the case study?

Is it to enable the course members to identify with some of the circumstances and realise through discussion that the issues are relevant and more than one solution is conceivable? Is it to enable members to learn to select information which is relevant to making decisions, to compare it with their own experience and disregard the rest? Is it to enable members either to reinforce or begin to change their attitudes?

Who is it for?

Is there some knowledge of the members' abilities? Have they been engaged in a similar exercise before? Is it important to include circumstances relating to particular ethnic groups, gender or marital status in the script?
Caution: It is easy to fall into the old trap of thinking that retirement is the domain of men (ie women neither work nor retire). Remember that people from various ethnic groups may differ in their perceptions of retirement.

What are the constraints?

Is there sufficient time available? Almost any case study will require at least an hour for the exercise and the summary. Is there sufficient space for the members to work in small groups?

What to include in the case study

- Decide on the overall length of the case study, the time it takes to read it and the main points you wish to emerge from the group discussion.
- List all the data you would like to include if you had unlimited space, then select the most important. If a piece from a government publication (eg a DSS leaflet) is to be used, consider its length and look out for technical terms or jargon.
- Decide how to use the less important material. Either forget it entirely and let the group members add anything they feel is important, or give additional material verbally as and when requested. Be consistent. Make certain the same information is available to all the participants.
- Make sure the facts are up-to-date. For example, DSS benefits change in November each year. If the case study is to be used during September to December insert 'Information accurate to November 1990' or a similar phrase.
- If the case study is fictitious make it credible. Group members will take the exercise seriously, and they will rightly feel indignant if they are presented with a 'larger than life' fairy tale.
- If what the case study describes is real and closely resembles an environment or setting with which the group members are familiar, the characters should be imaginary. In this instance it is crucial that none of the characters' names should be the same as any of the names of the group members.
- Present the written case study attractively and clearly.
- More information about the use of written case studies is on page 15.

Course Material

Topic A. Transition and time

This activity represents the step of the Coping with Change model, Identifying the Effects of Transition. Before the activity begins, draw a transition curve on the flipchart and write up the question (in italics below):

Activity

Ask the whole group '*What were your initial feelings about how your use of time might change when you first thought about retirement? Were they happy, apprehensive, mixed, exciting or challenging?*' Write up the comments made.
Allow 5-10 minutes for this.
When the list of comments is complete, discuss them in relation to the feelings of change plotted on the printed transition curve (Handout 1).
Allow 15 minutes for the whole of this activity.

Notes

Mention how this activity helps to set the scene for exploring the theme of time/structure. Participants may need some help in considering their reactions to the questions you have asked relating to their feelings, and especially to differentiate between those which are positive and those which are negative.

This activity allows participants to express negative feelings about changes (in retirement) if they choose. Acknowledge any comments of this nature even if they only come from one person. Be aware that within the group there may well be support for this person in the form of direct encouragement and others may relate similar personal experiences and describe ways in which they set about resolving issues.

Topic B. Analysis and use of time

B.1. Structure of time

In this activity participants move to the Taking Stock step of the Coping with Change model and consider the changes in the structure of time likely to be experienced by Jack and Mary (two of the characters in the Wyldes case study). Before you begin this activity, write up the questions (in italics below).

Activity

Option One

If this is the first time you have used the Wyldes case study, distribute Handouts 3a and 3b and either read them aloud or ask one of the participants to do so. Otherwise remind participants where they have used them before and ask them to glance through them again.

Divide participants into small groups and ask them to consider the questions:
What major differences in the structure of his time will Jack notice when he retires? What major differences in the structure of her time will Mary notice when Jack retires?
What constraints do you think Jack and Mary may be experiencing in the structure of their time in Jack's retirement?
What are the main points you would recommend Jack and Mary to consider when they discuss these changes?
Allow 15 minutes for this.

Then display the responses from each group on flipchart sheets, and/or invite comments on each question in turn.
Allow 20 minutes for this.

Option Two

This activity encourages participants to consider critically the structure and use of time by Jo and Billy (characters in the case study) before and after retirement, and corresponds to the Taking Stock part of the Coping with Change model. Handouts 4a and 4c describe the partners' timetables before retirement, and Handouts 4b and 4d describe their timetables after retirement. Write the questions (in italics below) on the flipchart paper before starting the activity.

Distribute Handouts 4a and 4c, weekly timetables for Jo and Billy before retirement, and divide participants into small groups. The following questions can be used to consider the issues in relation to the structure of time:
What do you notice about the time structure in Jo's life?
What do you notice about the time structure in Billy's life?
How much time do they spend in work?
How much time do they spend together?
How much space do they give (or allow) each other?

Now distribute Handouts 4b and 4d, after retirement, and ask:
What do you notice about the time structure in Jo's life now?
What do you notice about the time structure in Billy's life now?
How much time do they spend together?
How important is routine in their lives?
Are there any changes in the space they allow each other?
What are the main areas you would advise Jo and Billy to consider in relation to their use of time in retirement?
Discuss the changes which each of them have made.
Allow 30 minutes for this whole activity.

Notes	*All participants will acknowledge that away from paid work they will have more time to themselves 'to do the things I've always wanted to do' or 'to decide what I'm going to do with my time in the future'.*
	The activity in which they have considered the structure of time for the characters in either of the written case studies has not only reminded them of the number of hours given to work, but also that in retirement the consideration of the demands of the employer change to the considerations of the individual and the people with whom he or she lives. It is therefore important to be conscious of the way people quote themselves 'as the only person who now matters in the future use of time'.

Topic B. Analysis and use of time

B.2. Analysis of work

In this activity participants continue their consideration of the Taking Stock step of the Coping with Change model, thinking in terms of gains and losses in relation to the time spent in work (paid/unpaid). Participants are now encouraged to look at their own circumstances.

Activity

Ask participants. 'Try to estimate the amount of time you spend each day in work (including travel), either paid or unpaid. Then the amount of time in one week, one month and finally one year. Record these estimates on paper.'
'Now list the activities at work you find most enjoyable, and the amount of time spent on them per week.'
'Make a separate list of those activities at work you find least enjoyable, and state how much time each one takes up per week.'
Distribute Handout 5 and ask participants to complete it and discuss their answers with one other person.
Bring the group together again to compare experiences.
Allow 30 minutes for this activity.

Notes

When taking groups through these activities tutors should be aware of the status of individual participants with respect to the nature of work; paid'*work and/or work at home (housework), part-time paid work or voluntary work. It is also important to agree with the group on the use of the words 'work', 'employment' and unemployment. The simplest solution is to agree to use the word 'work', then add adjectives (such as paid/unpaid/voluntary) as appropriate. Unemployment is then the situation of a person who expects paid employment, but does not have it.*

In establishing the meaning of work mention the fact that many people spend more time in unpaid work than in paid work. Also draw attention to the part of life course spent in work, possibly as much as two-thirds. When inviting the group to think about the questions, say to the group 'Who is in control of your time now?', 'Who will be in control of your time when you retire?', 'How does this influence your reactions to this activity?' These activities can be especially helpful in considering the traditionally perceived roles of men and women in relation to paid and unpaid work, and the structures in work, either imposed or self-created, within which 'time' has been 'managed'.

B.3. Time management – what now?

This activity represents the Options and Choices steps of the Coping with Change model and provides an opportunity for participants to share information about current leisure activities.

Activity

At this point participants are invited to share their interests and leisure activities with the group. Use this opportunity to display information about local clubs and societies and opportunities for voluntary work.
Allow at least 3 minutes for each contribution.

Now ask the participants to consider individually 'What new interests/activities would I like to develop?' (Refer back to 'What do you want to do new?' in the Analysis of Work sheets). Participants can think about 'Do we mean *new* ones? Or have we always wanted to do them?' The answers can be put on their own sheets of paper under headings:
'New interests' i)   at home;
                 ii) outside the home.
After 5 minutes ask participants to put these in order of priority.
Now say 'For the first three priorities answer the following questions:

  How will I achieve this?
  Will there be any costs?
  Do I need anything else before I can achieve this?

After ten minutes ask the participants to find a partner to discuss these ideas, ie 'What I have always wanted to achieve is . . .' and 'The way I think I will achieve this is . . .'. After five minutes the other partner says what he or she would like to achieve. Ask the participants if they wish to share their ideas with the whole group.
Allow 20 minutes for this activity.

Notes

Use this activity as an opportunity for participants to hear about activities they may not have tried. In our experience most people are willing to share information about their interests but should not be over-persuaded.

This activity can result in individual participants committing themselves to a particular activity. The tutor or the group should not put pressure on them or be directive but should encourage people to express their intentions.

Themes of Change: Finance

Topics and method

A. Experience of financial change (tutor-led discussion)
B. Understanding personal finance
  B.1. Budgeting (case study: small group work – two options)
  B.2. Preparing a plan (case study: small group work)
  B.3. Identifying sources of help (case study: small group work)
  B.4. Using financial advisers (optional prepared question and answer session)
  B.5. The future (tutor's summing up)

Purpose

This theme is designed to simplify the terms and jargon associated with finance, to make participants more aware of their own skills in planning and managing finances, and to assist them in identifying and coping with both expected and unexpected changes in finance at this time. First, participants review their personal experience of change in financial status (Topic A) and then work on a task which draws on their own knowledge and encourages them to consider and identify the sources of advice and information they may need (Topic B). B.1–3 are continuous; each activity follows on from the one before. A case study is used to raise issues in a non-threatening way. By relating their own experience to the case study, participants are encouraged to compare views within the group. This exchange of opinions reinforces participants' awareness of the nature of the financial changes they have already experienced and the coping strategies they adopted then.

Options

The topics and activities are in sequence and take participants through most of the steps of the Coping with Change model. If other themes have been taken before this one, be aware of how links can be made to matters raised in other sessions. For instance: relationships – how partners need to plan together for the future; health – the need to budget for adequate nutrition; time – what using time profitably might mean. The

---

Information for tutors

Sources for reference are on page 68.

Practical points

Hints on how to use an outside speaker are on page 69.
Some notes on how to use a case study are on page 60.

Resources used in this theme

Flipchart, flipchart paper, pens, Blu-Tack
Handouts 3a and 3b: The Wyldes case study; 6: Wyldes budget checklist; 7: Personal budget checklist

Course material

Learning activities begin on page 70.
Handouts 3, 6 and 7 are on pages 105–106, 112–113.

Wyldes case study allows the issue of moving house to be explored. In Activity B.4 we have indicated where and how a financial adviser might be used, but the presence of an adviser is not essential.

Information for Tutors:

Sources for Reference

The course materials which follow are intended to help participants to formulate a positive way of thinking about anticipated changes in personal finance. In working through the steps of the model – in taking stock, identifying issues, in moving on to making choices – the process described helps participants to become aware of the information they will need in planning future action. The experienced tutor will build up a file of local contacts and resources. If time allows, expert opinion can be brought in as indicated in the text to deal with questions raised. The following titles indicate a starting point for reference for both tutor and participants.

Leaflets on pensions and other benefits are available from Post Offices or the local Department of Social Security offices. Freefone 0800 666555.

Notes of guidance on income tax are available from local tax offices or tax enquiry centres. Addresses are in the telephone directory under 'Inland Revenue'. (See especially leaflets IR 80, 81 and 91 for information about the independent taxation of women.)

Money Management Council, 18 Doughty Street, London W1N 2PL is a registered charity set up in 1985 to provide independent and impartial advice to promote a better understanding of personal and family finance. (NB The Council publishes information but does not offer individual or specific advice.)

Making a Will
Wills and Probate (Consumers Association, 1987).
Leaflets are available from Citizens' Advice Bureaux and Help the Aged.

The Time of Your Life (Help the Aged with the Health Education Council, first published 1979, many editions).

The State Pension Explained – A Guide for Women, by Barbara and Peter Spiers (GLAP, 1988).

Money, Your Rights and Retirement, by Edward Eaves (Choice, 1990).

Practical Points

While it is understandable that many (or even most) tutors may feel that their lack of knowledge of the world of finance will demonstrate their inadequacy in front of the group, it is important to distinguish between what the participants themselves know and wish to know, and what specific information or sources of information are available to meet those learning needs. This clearly demonstrates the problem-solving phase of the Coping with Change model.

Each participant will have acquired an enormous amount of practical experience over the years in managing his or her own money. Therefore it is worth identifying the aspects of finance which will change at retirement. For example, for some women the receipt of a state pension may signal a new phase in their lives, because they may not have received money 'in their own right' for a number of years. It is equally important to be aware of changes in financial legislation which affect everyone. Recent changes in the personal taxation of married women and the introduction of the Community Charge (poll tax) are two relevant examples.

Before using learning/teaching aids such as the Wyldes case study or budget sheets, check them for relevance to the participants, and update as necessary.

As recommended elsewhere, the benefits of working with other tutors can be substantial. For example, it may be possible to include a financial 'expert' in the team – one whose role in a more traditional pre-retirement course would have been to present a lecture based on a conventional syllabus. In this approach it is possible to work with the financial expert as a co-tutor, and to draw specifically on his or her particular expertise in response to group needs.

As a co-tutor the financial expert could, for example, sit in on the group discussion of the Wyldes' budgeting activity, design specific questions with you in order to engage the participants in meaningful discussion, take the feedback session, sit in as a member of a panel to respond to questions from the group and/or offer (or produce) relevant handout materials. Remember to allocate time for thorough preparation and rehearsal, if possible, beforehand, especially if a team-teaching approach is adopted.

Course Material

Topic A. Experience of financial change	This activity encourages participants to focus on the first step of the Coping with Change model, identifying the effects of transition.

Activity	Ask the question 'Can you recall when you first thought about financial changes as a result of your retirement? Can you recall your first feelings? Can you plot your feelings as they changed at particular ages or stages in your life?' Discuss the reactions from the group and use them to illustrate features of transition, such as the length of time (eg some participants may have identified their first thoughts of impending financial change five years or more before retirement), the nature of the transition, feeling able to cope, the 'peaks and troughs', when there seemed to be progress, and where they are along their own transition curve at present with regard to their personal finance. *Allow 25 minutes for this activity.*

Notes	*Changes in financial status are almost certain to happen to all people approaching retirement. The receipt of the state pension itself represents one (expected) change. While recognising the importance of the theme of finance, care should be taken not to 'isolate' it from other major themes of change or to exclude it from previous experience of handling change and assume it takes a special or unique place in preparing for retirement.*

Topic B. Understanding personal finance

B.1. Budgeting	This activity is concerned with the Identifying Issues step of the model. Two options are included. Using the budget sheet can enable participants to gain a sense of control over their

financial position and appreciate the options available in terms of changing expenditure.

Activity

Introduce the activity by asking the question 'What do we mean by budgeting? When we talk of people's financial affairs, what things do we include?' List the responses on a flipchart and include any important factors omitted (for instance, the value of property).

If this is the first time you have used the Wyldes case study, distribute Handouts 3a and 3b and either read them aloud or ask one of the participants to do so. Otherwise remind participants where they have used them before and ask them to glance through them again. Divide participants into small groups.

Option One
If you are using the budget sheets, also give out Handout 6 and ask 'What do you think you would do with the Wyldes' lump sum?' Participants then complete column two of the budget sheet.
Allow 45 minutes for this.

Option Two
If you are not using the budget sheet ask participants to identify the major financial issues the Wylde family face in the first year and agree the three most important financial issues.
Allow 15 minutes for this activity.

Notes

The case study is used to raise issues in a non-threatening way. By relating their own knowledge and skills to the case study, participants are encouraged to compare their own views within the group. This exchange of opinions reinforces the participants' awareness of the nature of the financial changes they have already experienced in life, and the coping strategy or strategies they have personally adopted during these periods. Because participants are encouraged to 'manage' the financial affairs of the Wyldes family in the case study, the whole exercise can generate lively discussion, laughter, moments of seriousness and an awareness that issues such as caring for others and perceived gender roles are often inextricably linked with a major change such as a financial one.

Follow on with B.2 immediately.

B.2. Preparing a plan

This activity leads naturally to preparing financial plans and is the Considering Options step of the Coping with Change model. The task of designing short- and medium-term strategies enables participants to draw heavily on their past experiences.

Activity	Invite participants, in the same groups, to use information from the previous activity and draw up financial plans for the Wyldes: short-term (one year) and medium-term (until Jack receives his state pension). Ask them to put their ideas on flipchart paper and then display the results. *Allow 20 minutes for this activity.*

Notes	*While participants are completing the tasks offer your support, for example, by asking questions like 'How might you overcome that financial issue you identified? What options or choices do you think are available?' People who live, or who have lived, on their own often demonstrate attitudes towards planning and skills in developing strategies which greatly enhance the group's task and learning. Finance tutors who may be participating in the group tasks will also find the group's opinions and ideas invaluable for later discussion.*

B.3. Identifying sources of help	This activity is a continuation of the previous work in B.1 and B.2 and the final step – the process of taking stock and considering the choices of the Coping with Change model – before taking action. It also represents the move from the case study, 'make-believe' approach to the actual 'live' situation, and demonstrates the value of the written case study in this process.

Activity	By referring to the issues arising from the financial planning task in the case study, make a list of all the sources of information and guidance needed to help in the planning process. Where possible identify the location either locally or nationally of each of these resources. *Allow 15 minutes for this.* Now ask participants 'Is there any information you need in your own financial planning that is different from what was identified in the case study?' *Allow 5 minutes here.*

Notes	*Encourage participants to identify in detail any support or help they think would be necessary. Identify areas where participants can themselves contribute information.*

B.4. Using financial advisers

Activity	Divide participants into small groups and ask them to draw up a list of questions they would want to ask a financial adviser to help them to develop their own financial plans. The groups can use information from the previous activities. After ten minutes, collate all the questions and check for clarity and possible duplication. Now put each question to the adviser(s) in turn. Allow time for additional comments or supplementary questions on the same issue from participants. Where new pieces of information or additional resources emerge, list these on a flipchart sheet for future reference. *Allow 25 minutes for this activity.*
Notes	*By collating the questions from the participants, it is possible to present the financial tutor(s) with two main tasks: to comment on the strategies recommended by the groups in relation to the case study; and to respond to the list of questions identified by the participants in the previous activities. This is also the opportunity to fill in any missing gaps specifically relevant to people approaching retirement. In this session, it is important to keep to an agreed time schedule. This may mean dividing the time available by the number of questions to be answered, allocating time for comment on the groups' strategies and for the summary comments. Any new information could be initially set out on a flipchart sheet and later typed and distributed to the participants.*
B.5. The future	This last activity provides the opportunity for participants to consider the Making Choices and Taking Action steps of the Coping with Change model and to reflect on their previous experiences, both in managing finance and in this programme.
Activity	Recap the stages of the Coping with Change model applied to finances. Now ask participants to take away with them and/or share with a partner, if they wish, their thoughts concerning the following: 'Remember the ways you have coped with financial change in the past; what steps will you take in handling your own personal financial position?' *Allow 5 minutes for this activity.*
Notes	*Participants are not expected to share their thoughts with the whole group. If you did not distribute the personal budget sheet (Handout 7) with your introductory letter, you could do so now.*

Themes of Change: Health

Topics and method

A. Health: what is it?
  - A.1. What does health mean? (trigger video or small group work)
  - A.2. Feelings about health (tutor-led discussion)
B. Health: taking charge
  - B.1. A review (tutor-led discussion of case study material)
  - B.2. Gains and losses (pair work followed by discussion)
  - B.3. Making health choices (optional use of health adviser)

Purpose

This theme is designed to relate to participants' own perceptions and expressed needs concerning health. Health is an integral concept of the Coping with Change model since any life change is likely to be accompanied by a change in health. Changes taking place at retirement can provide an opportunity for improvements in health. Participants are encouraged to look at the 'whole of health' rather than negatively at ill-health (Topic A); Topic B helps participants to identify options and choices in promoting their own health, consider sources of help and set realistic health goals.

Options

The topics and activities are sequenced and take participants through most of the steps of the Coping with Change model. If other themes have been taken before this one, be aware of how links can be made to matters raised in other sessions. For instance: relationships – doing things with other people promotes health; time – planning to use time in a way that stimulates the mind and the body; money – taking account of health needs when deciding where to economise. If moving house was raised, build in discussion about the desirability of avoiding too many stressful changes at once. In A.1 an alternative approach is suggested if video recording equipment is not available. A health adviser could be used in Topic B but is not essential to the course.

Information for tutors

Sources for reference are on page 75.

Practical points

Hints on how to use a trigger video are on page 76.

Resources used in this theme

Flipchart, flipchart paper, pens
Handouts 3a and 3b: The Wyldes case study; 8: Goal setting and health
Televison set, video recorder, CHRE video 'Focus on Health, Focus on Retirement'
What Next? Focus on Health, CHRE booklet

Course material

Learning activities begin on page 79.
Handouts 3 and 8 are on pages 105–106 and 114.

Information for Tutors:

Sources for Reference

The course materials which follow are intended to help participants to formulate a positive way of thinking about anticipated changes in health. In working through the steps of the model – in taking stock, identifying issues, in moving on to making choices – the process described helps participants to become aware of the information they will need in planning future action. The experienced tutor will build up a file of local contacts and resources. If time allows, expert opinion can be brought in as indicated in the text to deal with questions raised. The following titles indicate a starting point for reference for both tutor and participants.

Other CHRE publications:
Ideas and Resources for Health Educators, pack containing trigger video used in text.
What Next? – Focus on Health, booklet containing worksheet material for retirement groups.

Health Education Authority booklets:
A Guide to Healthy Eating
Exercise: Why Bother?

Better Health in Retirement, by J. A. Muir Gray (Age Concern, 1990).
The Time of Your Life (Help the Aged with the Health Education Council, first published 1979, many editions).

Other course material:
Health Education Authority – *Look After Yourself*
Open University – *Health Choices*; *Health and Retirement*

Practical Points

When to use a trigger video

- to introduce a theme or topic, or open the session
- at the end of a session, to consolidate the learning process
- to help the leader with little experience of group work who is learning to use the discussion method
- to create a climate for learning with a group which is slow to react or appears to need a stimulus
- to enable several small groups to work simultaneously.

Preparation

- When you are planning a session, decide what part the video will play.
- Make sure you are familiar with the equipment and that it is in working order.
- Preview the video (or part) you wish to use, time it and prepare any notes or handout materials.
- If possible, have the video recorder in position before the session, with the selected video ready for use.
- Try to remove any other displays or equipment which are likely to cause distraction.
- Plan how long the session will be and how the time will be allocated.

The CHRE video - 'Focus on Health, Focus on Retirement'

The CHRE video is divided into four parts. It can be used in a number of ways. In the first two examples given below, there are brief notes on how the video might be used, and the third is a more detailed example of the use of one person's reply to the question 'What does health mean to you?'

Example 1: 'What does health mean to you?'

Aim – to help participants to consider different ways of looking at health, what it is and what it means.
Objectives – to use the video as a means of engaging in dialogue with the group and identifying local facilities and sources of help in a wide range of health matters.

1. State reasons for using the video to the group and show it through without a break.
2. Follow up with a series of questions: 'Which particular comment is the one you most agree with?', 'Why?' and so on, and then 'Which particular comment on the video did you disagree with?', 'How do you think the person on the video felt when he or she made that comment?', 'Have you

ever felt like making the same comment yourself?', 'What do you think the facial expressions of the person making the comment were portraying?', 'Would you like to hear that comment again?'

3. Take the opportunity to move from general statements to the more specific. If someone agreed with the statement 'I really don't know how to judge health', you could find out how many other people in the group felt the same, then list the criteria on which 'health' could be judged. *Or if* someone quoted the comment 'Stress is a big killer', you could follow it up with your own question 'What do we mean by stress?'

4. Remember to allow time to achieve the second objective of identifying local health facilities and sources of help, and introduce this again with a question like 'Does anyone know if courses on managing stress are available locally?', or give information 'Do you know about the Look After Yourself courses held locally?'

5. Play the video through again in whole (or in part) if you and the group feel it will help to clarify your thoughts or refresh your memories.

Example 2: 'What are your thoughts on health and retirement?'

Aim – to prepare material for a debate, or questions for a panel, or brains trust, in a future health session.
Objective – to select some controversial statements which will form the basis for an exchange of views.

1. State your reasons for using the video.

2. Either use the whole video with the whole group or divide into four groups showing one part to each group. Allocate a number of comments for consideration. For example, *Comment 10. Part 4 (Diet)* 'I can only advise that in terms of full living and longevity you must watch your diet'. *Comment 13. Part 1 (Exercise)* 'I go through a phase of thinking I ought to be fit and make a half-hearted attempt at running around the park for a month and that never actually works out at all. Then I go back to hamburgers and stuff – then a month later I'll do the same again. So what happens is that I have a kind of paranoid approach to it that I must be fit but I don't actually do it.' *Comment 15. Part 2 (Self-employed)* 'Healthiest person I know? Mainly the old street traders [because] we have to be. If you're self-employed you cannot be ill.' *Comment 1. Part 3 (Concept of retirement)* 'I don't like the word.'

3. When enough relevant comments from the video have been selected, identify extra sources of materials which participants can consult locally or approach to build up the programme for the panel, brains trust or debate.

4. Remember to discuss outline programme(s) with other speakers taking part in the session as soon as possible and include selected comments from the video in the session itself.

Example 3: 'People seem to think that their health is the responsibility of doctors. This is something with which I totally disagree. We must be responsible for our own health.'

1. Show this comment (No. 26) from Part 1 to your group without any previous introduction of the topic. In other words let the video be the introduction.
2. Invite group members to say whether they agree or disagree with that statement. Take a vote, and quickly count the responses. (Remember to ask for Don't Knows.)
3. Invite the members to discuss the reasons for their responses to the statement in pairs.
4. Combine pairs into fours (or sixes if you are working with a total group of more than 12 people) and invite them to share with each other the views which were expressed in pairs.
5. Give these groups the additional task of summarising points both for and against the statement. Include areas unresolved by debate. Responses can be listed on flipchart sheets.
6. In the plenary session invite each group in turn (either through a spokesperson or collectively) to share the results of its discussion with the whole group, perhaps also answering questions.
7. There may be no need, or indeed any time, to summarise the main points of the discussion. On the other hand, you could consider the ways in which the issues which emerged from discussion could be developed during the rest of the course or after the course if the members so wish.

Example of action during the course

One of the main issues to emerge might be that of the doctor–patient relationship. 'I consider myself very lucky,' says one member. 'My doctor is excellent – he always makes time to listen, never fobs me off, and never questions if I want to call him if I'm ill.' 'That is certainly not my experience,' retorts another. 'You are herded into the waiting room, treated by the receptionist as though you cannot think for yourself and, when eventually you see the doctor, he is writing a prescription before he even looks up. What sort of service do you call that? I certainly only go to him if I have to, as a last resort.' Here is an opportunity for the group to role-play a short encounter between a doctor and a patient or to invite a general practitioner to join them on a future occasion for a discussion. Such an event can be useful to both parties. For example, the doctor and the group members might consider what each expects of the other: 'What do we expect from the doctor?' could be balanced by 'What are the doctor's expectations of the patients?'

Example of action outside (or after) the course

The group may have considered the original statement on the video too provocative. 'How is it possible to be responsible for our own health when work itself has damaged our health?' asks one member. 'I work in an unhealthy environment and I know my health has suffered because of my job. I go to the doctor to help me, but surely there is a responsibility on the part of employers and the government to help to create a healthy environment?'

If the group discussions have continued to develop this theme, they are beginning to consider important social issues and their relevance.

There is more information about using trigger videos on page 17.

Course Materials

Topic A. Health: what is it?

A.1. What does health mean?

This is the first activity within the health theme and sets the stage for an understanding of the meaning of health. It might be introduced by the use of the CHRE's trigger video or through discussion in small groups if the video is not available.

Before starting the activity write up the question (in italics below) on flipchart paper.

Activity

Begin by explaining that our thoughts about the meaning of health influence the health actions we take.

Option One
If the trigger video is used, ask participants 'Which of the statements made by people in the video do you agree with most? And which do you agree with least?' Show the video, divide participants into groups of about four and ask them to discuss the question *'So what does health mean to you now?'* After five minutes,

ask for comments from each group in turn and write them on flipchart paper. In summary identify the range of different interpretations of health, both positive and negative.
Allow 15 minutes for this.

Option Two
If the video is not used, begin by asking participants, in pairs, to consider the question '*Who is the healthiest person you know?*' After five minutes, combine pairs into groups of four to consider the question 'What does health mean to you now?' and proceed as above.
Allow 15 minutes for this activity.

Notes

This activity relates to the Taking Stock aspect of the Coping with Change model. Encourage participants to explore their understanding of the meaning of health; do not try to obtain a dictionary definition as this is unnecessary. Responses may lead to a summary in which health can be described as different stages of well-being, influenced by a person's physical, mental and social state. Encourage the group to end this short activity positively and lead straight into the next activity.

A.2. Feelings about health

In this activity participants consider their own feelings concerning health and well-being. In doing so they identify the changing nature of health and its relationship to the transition curve.

Activity

Say 'How do you know whether you are well or not? One simple test is to try concentrating on yourself for a few minutes. Nobody knows more about your health than you do. Do you feel well? Listen to your body. What is it telling you? How do you describe in words your feelings when you are really well?' Write up responses on the flipchart and discuss.

Now ask 'Do you think your experiences of health fit into the transition curve? Thinking about transitions you have experienced in life, is it possible to assess your health at different times in your life?' In the course of discussion point out that many factors affect people's health, including the work they have done, their housing conditions, whether they have lived in the country or the town, whether they are rich or poor. In your summing-up, say that almost anyone can, if they really want to, improve on their present level of health and increase their chances of staying healthy longer.
Allow 20 minutes for this activity.

Notes	*Do not force your own interpretations of the meanings of health which participants identify. The most important features of this activity are that participants recognise that we feel we know when we have good health but that it is difficult to describe, and that almost everyone can, if they wish, improve their present health status.*
	(This activity and those which follow can be amplified by using material from the CHRE booklet What Next? – Focus on Health. *This would be an appropriate time to distribute copies of the booklet and invite participants to discuss the text with their partners and/or other members of their families at their leisure.)*

Topic B. Health: taking charge

B.1. A review

This activity encourages participants to focus on the Identifying Issues step of the Coping with Change model. Prepare for this activity and the one which follows by marking two columns on a flipchart sheet, one headed Case Study 'Health Reducing' and the other Case Study 'Health Improving'.

Activity

If the Wyldes case study has been used before, remind participants about it and ask them to glance through it again. If this is the first time you have used it, distribute copies (Handouts 3a and 3b) and either read them out loud or ask one of the participants to do so. Introduce the activity to participants by asking 'Can you find examples in the case study of behaviour which is both health improving and health reducing?'

Using flipchart paper write up the health improving and reducing activities or factors identified by participants. Be prepared to discuss any areas of disagreement or uncertainty.
Allow 30 minutes for this activity.

Notes

This activity encourages participants to focus on the wide range of activities/factors which influence health, some of which may not have been considered before. It is important to consider the idea that changes at this time of life may improve *health, if this has not been mentioned before.*

B.2. Gains and losses

This activity is a continuation of B.1 and moves on to the problem-solving phase of the model. Prepare a sheet of flipchart paper marking two columns, one headed 'Health Reducing' and the other 'Health Improving'.

Activity

Introduce the activity by saying, 'I said just now that health can be improved at any age. Do you agree with this statement? In the past who decided about your health? Who decides now? How far are we really able to make choices about our own health?'

Now ask participants, in pairs, to discuss and write down aspects of their own lives which they consider (1) health improving and (2) health reducing. Consider this question in the context of paid work, unpaid work, leisure and social activities and so on.
Allow 10 minutes for this.

Bring the groups together and collate the lists of health reducing and health improving responses. Discuss these, inviting clarification where necessary. Relate the activity to the Coping with Change model. Discuss the opportunities retirement may bring to improve health.
Allow 15 minutes for this.

Notes

Ageism and social attitudes have promoted (often invalid) views on the decline of health with age; health can be improved at any age. Participants may or may not be prepared to recognise aspects of their own lives which influence health.

B.3. Making health choices

In this activity participants are invited to plan action they might take to improve their health, the Making Choices step of the Coping with Change model. An option here might be to have a health adviser present to comment on and add to participants' ideas and goals.

Activity

Ask participants to return to their pairs from the previous activity and identify the way they will seek to influence their own health in the short term (six months) and medium term (one year). Distribute Handout 8 goal setting and health to help with this process.
Allow 15 minutes for this activity.

Ask the whole group if there are any points wish to raise. Sum up this series of exercises by pointing out that participants have considered their own lives and how they can improve their own health by taking certain actions.
Allow 15 minutes for this.

Notes

The purpose of writing down possible action is to help participants to identify the individual steps they can take to improve their health. If a visiting expert is there to comment on participants' plans, ensure enough time is allocated for discussion based on participants' plans.

Themes of Change: Relationships

Topics and method

A. Transition and relationships
B. Changing relationships
    B.1. Close relationships (trigger video or case studies followed by tutor-led discussion)
    B.2. Options and strategies (case study, small group discussion with leader, report)
    B.3. Communication – what do I say now? (small group discussion, report back)
    B.4. Negotiation – wanting different things (whole and small group work)
    B.5. Emotion – I feel . . . will you? (whole group and paired work)

Purpose

This theme aims to help participants to come to terms with the fact that one of the unavoidable implications of retirement concerns changes in patterns of relationships in both work and non-work environments, and to encourage participants to identify skills they feel might be helpful in developing and maintaining relationships. First, participants explore feelings around changing relationships (Topic A); they then consider issues concerning various types of prejudice (Topic B) and go on to identify how retirement can influence close relationships.

Options

The topics and activities are sequenced and take participants through most of the steps of the Coping with Change model. If other themes have been taken before this one, be aware of how links can be made to matters raised in other sessions. For instance: time – the need to negotiate with others how time is spent; money – again the need to negotiate with others in planning a budget: see activities B.1 and B.2; health – how loneliness can become a health problem. If moving house was an issue raised, build in discussion about the need to negotiate all major changes with others involved. There are a number of options: in B.1 if a video is not available two case studies can be used; in B.2 two alternative case studies are presented.

Information for tutors

Sources for reference are on page 85.

Practical points

Notes for using the 'Retired Not Out' video are on page 86.

Resources used in this theme

Flipchart, flipchart paper, pens
Notepaper, pencils
Handouts 3a and 3b: The Wyldes case study; 4a–d: Timetables, before and after retirement; 9: I feel . . . will you?
Television set, video recorder and the video 'Retired Not Out'

Course material

Learning activities begin on page 86.
Handouts 3, 4 and 9 are on pages 105–110 and 115.

If participants wish to extend this programme Topics B.3–5 can be used to consider strategies which may be helpful in communication, negotiation and expression of feelings.

Information for Tutors:	# *Sources for Reference*

The course materials which follow are intended to help participants to formulate a positive way of thinking about anticipated changes in relationships. In working through the steps of the model – in taking stock, identifying issues, in moving on to making choices – the process described helps participants to become aware of the information they will need in planning future action. The experienced tutor will build up a file of local contacts and resources. The following titles indicate a starting point for reference for both tutor and participants.

Black and Ethnic Minority Elders – Retirement Issues, by Ferdinand Fru and Frank Glendenning (PRA, 1989).
Games People Play, by Eric Berne (Penguin Books, 1964).
I'm OK You're OK, by A. and T.M. Harris (Pan Books, 1969).
People Skills: How to Assert Yourself, Listen to Others, and Resolve Conflict, by R. Bolton (Spectrum, Prentice Hall Inc, New Jersey, 1979).
Taking Stock: Being Fifty in the Eighties, by Charles Handy (BBC Publications, 1983).
The Time of Your Life (Help the Aged with the Health Education Council, first published 1979, many editions).
What Every Woman Should Know about Retirement, by Helen Franks (Age Concern, 1987).
A Woman in Your Own Right: Assertiveness and You, by A. Dickson (Quartet, 1982).

Practical Points

We suggest that tutors consider using the video 'Retired Not Out' developed by Learning in Later Life (1981–89), a programme for retired people at North London Polytechnic. The video is obtainable from the Administrator, Access and Community Centre, Room 112, North London Polytechnic.

The video portrays issues around ageism, sexism, and stereotyed roles.

Example: Video sequence: people talking on a bus journey

Aim – to help participants to identify bias and prejudice concerning ageism in everyday situations.
Objectives – to use the video as a means of engaging in dialogue with a group on the sensitive issues of ageism and sexism.

1. Play the video sequence without explanation to participants.
2. Follow up with a series of questions: 'What did you see happening in the video?', 'Why do you think the male passenger behaved like he did?', 'What does this tell you about his attitudes to age and women over 60?', 'How do you think the female passenger may have felt?'
3. 'In what other ways could the conversations have been developed?'
4. 'If you were re-making this video, how would you write the script to overcome the prejudices the actors portrayed?'

Course Material

Topic A. Transition and relationships

This is the first step of the Coping with Change model. Participants are encouraged to identify the way they feel in anticipation of changing relationships in retirement. Draw the transition curve on the flipchart before you begin this activity.

Activity	Introduce the theme by relating back to its initial selection. Say 'Looking at the transition curve in relation to people you associate with at work, can you think of one person (or several) whose company you will miss? What words may express some of your feelings about these changes?' Invite them to share this information with another person in the group if they wish. *Allow 10 minutes for this.*
	In the whole group invite participants to bring out any points they felt were important to them when doing this exercise. *Allow 10 minutes for this activity.*

Notes	*When participants describe changing friendships, indicate that this has involved both 'letting go' and 'continuing' some friendships. Encourage participants to acknowledge the 'gains' and 'losses' in this process. Be sensitive to participants' responses: some feelings mentioned may be associated with major losses in their lives.*

Topic B. Changing relationships

B.1. Close relationships	This activity corresponds to the Taking Stock step of the Coping with Change model. Three options are described, one using a video and two using case studies, to explore these relationships. Use the discussions to encourage participants to identify how far their own and others' attitudes may limit perceptions of options or choices.

Activity	**Option One**
	If the Wyldes case study has been used before, remind participants about it and ask them to glance through it again. If this is the first time you have used it, distribute Handouts 3a and 3b and either read them aloud or ask one of the participants to do so. Divide the participants into groups of four and ask them to discuss the following: *'How may relationships change for characters in the case study?'*
	Suggest that they might consider the following: relationship changes at work, ie in paid, unpaid and voluntary work; relationship changes in the non-work environment, ie home (the people we live with) and clubs, churches etc. *Allow 15 minutes for this.*
	Now ask about each of the characters: *Who do you think are the powerful characters? Why?*

Who do you think is independent? Who do you think is dependent? Why do you think this?
What assumptions have you made about the characters in the case study? Are there other interpretations? If so, what conclusions may you draw now?
Did all the members of your group think the same way?

Then ask participants 'What issues, concerns or problems do you think these characters could face with respect to these changes?' Now ask the group to display their flipchart sheets. Review the changes and the range of issues identified by participants in the whole group.
Allow 35 minutes for this.

Option Two
Distribute Handouts 4a–d. Divide participants into groups of four and ask them to discuss the following: '*In what ways may relationships change for characters in the case study?*'
Suggest that they might consider the following: relationship changes at work, ie in paid, unpaid and voluntary work; relationship changes in the non-work environment, ie home (the people we live with) and clubs, churches etc.
Allow 15 minutes for this.

Then ask participants 'What issues, concerns or problems do you think these characters could face with respect to these changes?' Now ask the group to display their flipchart sheets. Review the changes and the range of issues identified by participants in the whole group.
Allow 25 minutes for this.

Option Three
Show the video 'Retired Not Out' (see Practical Points) and ask participants to consider the following:
Who do you think are the powerful characters? Why?
Who do you think is independent? Who do you think is dependent? Why do you think this?
What assumptions have you made about the characters in the case study? Are there other interpretations? If so, what conclusions may you draw now?
Did all the members of your group think the same way?
What views appear to be expressed about ageism and sexism?
How do you think the characters felt because of the way they were addressed?
If you were re-writing the sketch for the video, what changes would you make?
Obtain feedback and discuss the issues raised by the participants.
Allow 20 minutes for this activity.

Notes

Option One. When dividing the group, suggest they concentrate on different characters in the case study. Make sure all characters are included. Emphasis on certain characters may be needed because of the backgrounds and experiences of your group, ie a large number of single people, or a particular ethnic mix. When a character in the case study is considered, ask participants to put themselves in that person's place and see the world from his or her point of view.

The questions are designed to encourage participants to consider the way they think about age, people's roles and relationships. While the activity is going on circulate round the groups listening and offering comments or prompts as necessary.

Be aware that people of any age may have negative attitudes to people older or younger than themselves.

Option Two. *These case studies allow consideration of complex relationship issues through a relatively simple timetable format. The case study has been developed so that assumptions made by participants can be explored. These may include: the nature of the partnership – married, cohabiting, homosexual or heterosexual; age; and people's roles and relationships. While the activity is going on circulate round the groups listening and offering comments or prompts as necessary.*

Be aware that people of any age may have negative attitudes to people older or younger than themselves.

Option Three. *The different scenarios in the video are humorous but carry an underlying serious message.*

B.2. Options and strategies

This activity leads directly on from B.1 and corresponds to the Choices and Options steps of the Coping with Change model. In this activity participants will identify the possibilities available to characters in the case study.

Activity

Ask participants to identify and list the options open to the characters to maintain or develop relationships with each other. Say 'How do you suggest they do this? What might be the consequences of these changes and for whom?' After 20 minutes the groups display their flipchart sheets. Discuss the options and strategies participants suggest.
Allow 35 minutes for the whole activity.

Notes

If participants suggest that certain characters in the script should get together and talk through problems, this will be an opportunity for you to point out that 'talking more' may be an over-simplistic view when compared to real life. Activities B.3–7 are optional and can be used to provide an opportunity for participants to consider the way they communicate, negotiate and express their feelings.

B.3. Communication - what do I say now?

This activity identifies a way of taking action and relates to an extension or development of that step of the model. Adopt an appropriate example from the Wyldes case study (Handouts 3a and 3b).

Activity

If this is the first time the case study has been used, either read it aloud or ask one of the participants to do so. Otherwise remind the participants about it and ask them to glance through it again. In this activity participants will be asked to complete a conversation on behalf of one of the characters. Set the scene by identifying that Jack will be retiring in six months and lives with Mary. Make the statement clearly but without emotion, ie neither sad nor happy; do not say the words casually. Say, 'One of the partners, Mary, says, "I don't really want to retire when you do."' Each participant now writes down what Jack says in reply to Mary. When all participants have completed their responses, write up their answers on flipchart paper.

Divide participants into groups of four and ask them to say: Which comments/answers close up the conversation and why do they do this? Which comments/answers open up the conversation?

Discuss the answers from each group and write the main points on the flipchart.
Allow 35 minutes for this activity.

Notes

Write up all the answers from the first part of the activity whether they appear to be serious or not. Participants may make particular suggestions in their groups which relate to good communication and listening skills, such as looking at Mary, listening to what and how words are said and by being attentive; and by comments like 'yes' or ' I see' to indicate understanding of a point of view or piece of information.

Open-ended questions require the person to expand on or add to what he or she has already said. Closed questions can be answered with a 'yes' or 'no', or even with a flippant remark such as 'Wasn't it a sunny day today!'

B.4. Negotiation - wanting different things

This is a further activity which helps participants to practise ways of getting the most out of the process of negotiation with a partner. This example is taken from the Wyldes case study. Before starting the activity write the questions (in italics below) on the flipchart.

Activity	Present the situation where Mary would like Marion to encourage her mother to make a will. Working in pairs, discuss the following questions adopting the roles of a) Mary and b) Marion in turn: *What will you do before you start to negotiate?* *Is it important to be prepared?* *How will you approach the conversation with Mary/Marion?* *What will be the best outcome to aim for?* *What is the minimum you will be prepared to accept in this negotiation?* *How would you negotiate in this position?* *Allow 15 minutes for this.* Now engage participants in open discusion using volunteer 'pairs' to share the results of their role-play, and what they have learned from this activity. *Allow 25 minutes for the whole activity.*
Notes	*Very little information is given in the case study about the thoughts or concerns of either Mary or Marion in relation to Mother's will. Therefore the success of the activity depends to a great extent on the experience and skills of the participants.*
B.5. Emotion - I feel . . . will you?	In this activity participants (using the case study) can consider a number of ways people express their feelings when engaged in negotiations; for example, without being over-assertive or blaming another. Before the activity begins, ensure you are familiar with the material.
Activity	Participants continue to work in their pairs from activity B.4. Distribute Handout 9: I feel . . . will you? and read it through to participants. Then invite them to recall any part of their role-play negotiations that produced a particular reaction or emotion. Now refer to the example and notes of guidance, on the handout, and with a partner work through and record responses to the first four phrases. *Allow 15 minutes for this.* Invite the whole group to discuss the value of this activity and its application to real life. *Allow 30 minutes for the whole activity.*
Notes	*The strategy outlined in Handout 9 is recommended as a way of avoiding accusation and blame. Steps 1–3 'When you . . .', 'I felt . . .' and 'because . . .' can be used on their own. In this form they allow a person to assert his or her own feelings linked to someone else's perceived*

behaviour. Step 4 'Will you . . .' can be added, but emphasise the need for care. During the paired activity participants may experience the feelings of the role. These feelings can be helpful in developing an understanding of other people. In the discussion of the phrases and paired work ask participants to share their thoughts and feelings about this technique and its possible use.

Review – The Final Session

Stages and method

10. Review of major themes and issues (tutor-led discussion)
11. Evaluation (questionnaire)
12. What next? (open forum)

Purpose

In this session the tutor and participants review the whole programme (Stage 10), determine to what extent the main aims have been achieved (Stage 11), and consider possible ways forward (Stage 12).

Options

Stage 12 will take a variety of forms, but will offer participants the opportunity to discuss the possibility of meeting again.

Information for tutors

Some notes on evaluation are on page 94.

Practical points

Further thoughts on running this session are on page 95.

Resources used in Stages 10-12

Flipchart, flipchart paper, pens
Flipchart sheets compiled in earlier sessions
Tape recorder
Handout 10: evaluation form

Course material

Learning activities begin on page 96.
Handout 10 is on page 116.

Information for Tutors:	*Evaluation*

Both the teacher and the learner are inextricably linked in the assessment. 'Because education involves human interaction, all personal criticism, whether it is the teacher criticising the learner, or the learner criticising the teacher, should be undertaken sensitively, recognising once again that the criteria for evaluation are personal and subjective, and that the human being receiving the criticism is both unique and invaluable' (P. Jarvis, *Professional Education*, Croom Helm, 1983).

Evaluating educational experiences at the end of a course or programme is notoriously difficult and not particularly reliable. However, there are at least three specific areas which may be considered systematically: the purpose (of the event), its content (ie the curriculum) and its methodology. Each participant will have his or her own ideas or criteria on which to base evaluation of any or all of these areas.

To a large degree these assessments will be subjective; for example, participants may well be comparing the tutor with a schoolteacher of some 40 years ago. On the other hand, evaluation of the content of the programme may be undertaken objectively. Participants can refer back to their flipchart summaries, and consider whether each theme or item within each theme has been covered; its relative value to each individual as well as to the group as a whole; and to what extent too much or too little time was spent on exploring that item. Understanding the various issues or items of fact must, however, be subjective. Because the participants themselves have been engaged in the process of determining the content, their criteria for evaluation must necessarily include their own individual contributions to the group.

There are further notes on evaluation on page 25 and in Appendix 2.

Practical Points

There should be certain features of this 'ending' of the programme which distinguish its uniqueness, focusing on the extent of the participants' involvement and the role taken by the tutor. If the initial aims were set out clearly by the tutor and shared by the participants, this session should reflect recognisable elements of joint learning and shared 'ownership' of the whole programme. Examples of this will be seen from the willingness of individuals to adopt 'leadership' roles when, for example, giving specific information to the whole group, drawn either from their own experiences or research for this event, or both. Equally, the tutor's reactions both to accepting such temporary changes in roles and to harnessing such group experiences are clear indications of the developmental nature of the programme in practice and its acknowledgement by all the members. On some occasions, being a part of this process may be difficult for some tutors, for traditionally the continued reliance on the 'expert' knowledge of the tutor can be interpreted as personally 'rewarding', whereas the observable movement towards greater autonomy (in thinking, understanding the process, and 'owning' the curriculum) on the part of the participants may lead a tutor to ask 'What have I been doing and what has been my role?'

To reflect on such questions may, in itself, lead to a greater understanding of the process in which the participants themselves have been engaged, also to the development or enhancement of the skill which Knowles (*The Modern Practice of Adult Education*, Associated Press, Chicago, 1970) described as enabling the tutor to 'suppress his own compulsion to teach what he knows his students ought to learn in favour of helping his students learn for themselves what they want to learn'.

Course Material

Stage 10. Review of major themes and issues

In these final stages participants and tutor review and evaluate the programme. In this stage participants are invited to reconsider their thoughts about retirement prior to coming on the programme, and then to review the effects of considering their experiences of change and transition in the context of retirement. This leads to a review of the priorities set by participants, the rationale and approach of the programme and whether needs have been met.

Ensure the flipchart sheets compiled in Stages 8 and 9 are displayed.

Activity

Introduce this activity, suggesting the way it could be developed and ask participants, 'What did you think about starting with the meaning of retirement? How did this help you to focus on your experiences of life changes?'

Through a series of questions and/or comments made during this discussion, explain your reasons for beginning this exercise with the analysis of change. Invite participants to comment on what differences (if any) they would have experienced if the whole programme had started with the analysis of change rather than with an exploration of the meaning of retirement. Discuss the extent to which the group now feels that the coping with change process requires a sound understanding of life changes and the experiences of transition.

Now invite participants to look back at the flipchart sheets they drew up on the themes of change (Stages 8–9) and review how the approach adopted contributed to their understanding and involvement. Before you complete this stage check that all the issues raised have been covered, either in group work or by individual comment.

Allow 45 minutes for the whole activity.

Notes

During the process of reviewing the programme participants may raise questions of fact which they hope will have immediate answers. The temptation for the tutor to answer all the questions to 'the best of his or her ability' is great; a wiser approach is to invite responses from other group members, and also to identify (if possible) reliable sources of information.

In the light of the group's understanding of the Coping with Change model, review the two dimensions involved in each step of the process: meaning (including understanding, knowledge and, to some extent, content) and involvement (including feelings, planning and learning). For example, in the theme of finance, participants can decide their own current position in the transition process by assessing their understanding and actions taken (or anticipated) in relation to some issues, yet realise that they have to go through a similar process with other issues to enable them to complete the transition process successfully. One of the results of this exercise is the realisation that the major themes of change are interwoven into the 'fabric of life' and the coping (or managing) process crosses and re-crosses all those boundaries, though some 'themes' are more dominant or complete than others for some individuals. As each theme is reviewed, refer to the list of sources available for further help or information. Also check that the relevant handout materials have been distributed.

Stage 11. Evaluation

Explain your reasons for conducting this activity and say what you mean by words like evaluation and assessment.

Activity

There are many ways of obtaining feedback from the group, and it is suggested that either or both of the following methods will be effective.

1. Distribute a questionnaire (Handout 10) to each participant and allow sufficient time for completion. Be prepared to accept that some people will not wish to do this part of the evaluation exercise. Try not to be too directive or meticulous about the completion of the questionnaires, and encourage people to work on their own or in pairs if this is more acceptable. At the end of this part of the task, ask the participants if they have any particular comments about the programme which they are willing to state openly and record on tape. *You must have their agreement to record their comment.* Experience has shown that it is sometimes useful to focus the question more sharply, for example, by taking each of the major themes in turn. Refer back to Stage 10 if a very open form of assessment took place during the review process.

2. A second method of obtaining feedback involves dividing the participants into groups of four and asking them to identify no more than five aspects/features of the course which they found most helpful or in which they were conscious that new learning had taken place. A flipchart can be used. After 10–15 minutes, invite each small group to share their comments with the whole group and engage in 'question and answer' and/or discussion around any area as necessary. With the agreement of the group, record this session on tape.
Allow 35 minutes for the whole activity.

Notes

The questionnaires are particularly useful in that they allow participants to focus on the parts of the programme where they have strong interests or opinions and to express their opinions on paper. This written expression can be a helpful complement to the spoken opinion in assessment and evaluation.

The questionnaires are also an important contribution to the tutor's understanding of individual priorities and reactions to the programme. They will probably reflect both the similarities and differences of other groups engaged in a similar programme and certainly add to the tutor's experience of working with groups.

On some occasions, certain written comments may be usefully fed back to the employer or funding agency to assist, for example, in their understanding of participants' needs and the relevance of their own policies towards such programme provision.

Stage 12. What next?

This stage in the programme will take different forms according to circumstances. Here are some examples.

If the participants are employed by the same company which offers post-retirement facilities and/or benefits, an employer representative could explain what is available at this point, and distribute appropriate literature.

Similarly, if the tutor has a welfare role in the organisation, details of individual support available until and, where applicable, into retirement can be fully explained to the participants.

Occasionally, even in a group from a variety of employers, information can be given about the location and contacts of the local or regional representative of the retirement fellowship, and whether such membership extends to friends or associates from other companies. For example, the Civil Service and the National Health Service have a national network of post-retirement fellowships and a central contact for information.

The participants may wish to meet together again in, say, a year's time. Here the tutor should encourage the spokesperson (there usually is one) who has initiated the idea to 'chair' the group while this debate is proceeding. It is also helpful to encourage the group to make certain decisions here. For example, one person may volunteer to contact all those who are interested. Names and addresses can be exchanged straightaway and a date arranged (with a venue) for the reunion meeting. On some occasions the tutor is also involved, but this is not necessarily always the case or even desirable.

This session can be very successful and an excellent example of good adult education practice, where the leadership role is taken by a participant or in turn by a number of participants, and the tutor adopts a participative, observing role.

Experience shows that the time allowed for the whole of this final session varies from 45 minutes to 2 hours 30 minutes.

Handout Sheets 1 - 10

Coping with change - a pattern of transition

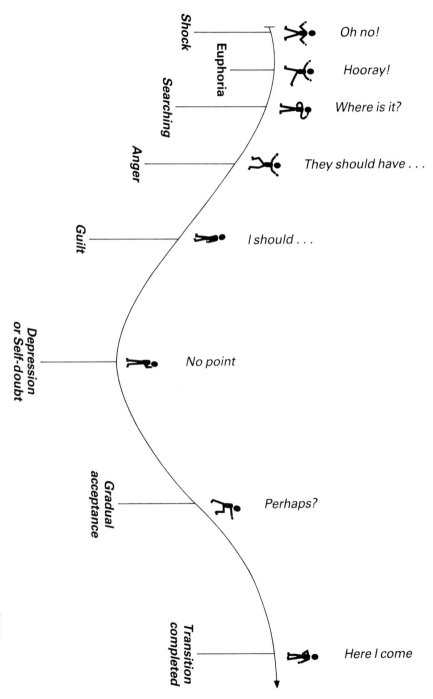

Coping with Change model

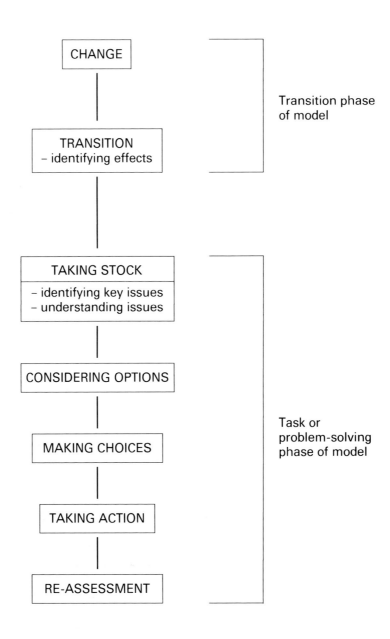

© CHRE 1991

Case study: the Wyldes

Jack is 62 and Mary 61. They have their own semi-detached house in Mansfield and have completed the mortgage payments. The house is situated on a steep hill overlooking the town. They have one daughter who lives about two and a half miles away. She is married and has three daughters. Mary was an only child. Her mother died some years ago and her father now lives in a home for the elderly in Birmingham. Jack has one sister, Marion, who is not married and has just retired. For more than 20 years she has worked and lived in hotels in London. Marion has bought a small flat near her friends in Blackpool with whom she spends a lot of time. She feels she will be financially secure and looks forward to her life in retirement.

Jack has worked for the same company for 34 years and has decided to leave in August when he will be 63. He does a lot of walking and climbing of stairs at work and feels pretty fit, although he actually hates walking. To his surprise he recently discovered that he walked an average of 11 miles a day at work but complains that his feet and legs ache quite a lot. He will be pleased not to have to do all that walking and will use the car more to get about as he gets older. Jack only uses the car on his days off and at weekends and then mainly for shopping and visiting the grandchildren and his mother.

Mary doesn't drive and for the last ten years she has walked the three-quarters of a mile to and from the bus stop three times a week to get to her part-time job. Mary does not get a pension from her job. Jack wants her to leave her job when he retires. She doesn't really want to but on the other hand she is looking forward to getting around in the car – no more long walks in all weathers to the bus stop.

They were very surprised when they recently added up their savings (not counting any lump sums, but including an insurance policy which matures when Jack is 65) and found they came to £11,000 plus the value of the house. However, Jack did wonder whether he really should get another job to take him over 65. Jack will receive a pension of £3,300 plus a lump sum of £9,900 from his employer when he is 63.

He fancies a bungalow in Farnsfield to be nearer his widowed mother. Mother is 88 years old and lives on her own in a two-bedroomed bungalow with a large garden. She is very active but does find the garden too much and hates shopping in the supermarket. She relies heavily on Jack and Mary for company and help with her gardening and shopping.

At her 80th birthday party Mother announced her wish to Marion, Jack and Mary that after her days Jack should have the bungalow, and Marion, Jack and Mary should share all her other possessions between them and sell anything they don't want.

Mary doesn't like this idea very much because she knows that her mother hasn't made a will, but won't say anything because she is, after all, an in-law.

Mary has that niggling feeling that Jack's mother will become more demanding when Jack finishes work and in her heart Mary doesn't want to move from the house which holds so many happy memories for all the family.

Case study: Marion Wylde

Marion is 60 years of age and is experiencing her first year in retirement in a completely different environment from the hotel staff accommodation she had been in for more than 20 years.

Marion was quite close to Jack until he married and then whenever they met up Marion stayed with their mother in her bungalow.

Mary and Jack's grand-daughters always enjoy aunty Marion's very occasional visits, especially Katie, who is just 13 years old and would love to leave home and work in an hotel like Marion.

Marion never glamorises her job in front of Katie, for she still recalls her own childhood, when she felt that she was expected to do far more things about the house than Jack and it was made pretty clear to her when she was about 14 years old that Jack's further education in the local technical college was 'more important for a boy than a girl'. She was never consciously jealous of Jack, but he seemed more close to their mother and Marion to their father, especially when she was a teenager.

She left school at 15 with a very good report in needlework, cookery and pottery and obtained her job with a large group of hotels by answering an advertisement in a national paper. Over the years she did most jobs in an hotel and progressed far beyond her wildest expectations and even refused on several occasions to take a position as manageress.

She has a small circle of friends with whom she feels particularly at ease, and most of these she has met during the last ten years. Many of the earlier friendships caused her some embarrassment and inward 'frustration' especially with those who 'expected' her to be married by 25, then by 30, and seemingly would not accept that her thoughts on close relationships with friends of both sexes were highly personal. She can recall only one occasion when, in a moment of temper, she actually disclosed that she had refused 'more than one' offer of marriage.

At present, life seems pretty good for Marion, and she is still quite euphoric about the normal life she is leading as opposed to her usual unsocial and unpredictable hours on duty in the hotel. Retirement is with her and she has tackled the first hurdle by finding a home – anything else she'll just take as it comes.

A timetable: before retirement

Jo

	Monday	Tuesday	Wednesday	Thursday	Friday	Saturday	Sunday
Morning	Work	Work	Work	Work	Work	Garden	Clean car Read Sunday papers Pub
Afternoon	Work	Work	Work	Work	Work	Watch TV sport	lunch Drive
Evening	Watch TV	Have drinks with workmates	Shopping	Watch TV	Have drinks with workmates	Visit family	Watch TV

Billy

	Monday	Tuesday	Wednesday	Thursday	Friday	Saturday	Sunday
Morning	Work	Work	Work	Work	Work	Washing Housework	Housework Pub
Afternoon	Visit parents	Shopping	Housework	Reading	Swimming	Reading Ironing	lunch Drive
Evening	Social secretary work	Pottery class	Shopping	Letter writing	Watch TV	Visit family	Watch TV

© CHRE 1991

A timetable: after retirement

Jo

	Monday	Tuesday	Wednesday	Thursday	Friday	Saturday	Sunday
Morning	Nothing	Shopping	Nothing	Gardening Pub	Nothing	Gardening	Clean car Pub
Afternoon	Watch TV	Nothing	Watch TV	Lunch Library Reading	Nothing	Visit family	lunch Drive
Evening	Watch TV	Social club	Clean windows	Watch TV	Pub Watch TV	Watch TV	Watch TV

Billy

	Monday	Tuesday	Wednesday	Thursday	Friday	Saturday	Sunday
Morning	Housework	Shopping	Visit friends	Gardening Pub	Ironing Housework	Relaxed morning	Read Sunday papers Pub
Afternoon	Visit parents	Swimming	Pottery class	Lunch Cooking	Swimming	Visit family	lunch Drive
Evening	Social secretary work	Social group	Watch TV	Letter writing	Watch TV	Watch TV	Watch TV

A timetable: before retirement (single person)

	Monday	Tuesday	Wednesday	Thursday	Friday	Saturday	Sunday
Morning	Work	Work	Work	Work	Work	Washing Shopping	Religious assembly Housework
Afternoon	Work	Work	Work	Work	Work	Gardening	Visit relatives
Evening	Letter writing Watch TV	Evening class pottery	Clean car Reading	Housework	Theatre or concert or entertain friends	Ironing Watch TV	Watch TV Reading

© CHRE 1991

A timetable: after retirement (single person)

	Monday	Tuesday	Wednesday	Thursday	Friday	Saturday	Sunday
Morning	Housework	Shopping Washing	Ironing	Housework	Gardening	Lazy start	Religious assembly
Afternoon	Letter writing	Cooking	Visit friends	Clean car	Reading/ library	Visit friends	Visit relatives
Evening	Reading Watch TV	Evening class pottery	Visit friends/ watch TV	Nothing	Theatre or concert or entertain friends	Watch TV	Watch TV

© CHRE 1991

Analysis of work		
Things/facets of work you are happy to leave behind	Things/facets of work you wish to 'take over' into retirement	Things in life you would like to start new in your retirement

The Wyldes case study:

budget checklist

	Year before retirement £	*Year after retirement* £

INCOME
    Wages/salary (including part-time earnings)
    State retirement pension (and graduated pension)
    Occupational pension
    Other income (eg investment interest etc)

TOTAL INCOME (gross)

EXPENDITURE

    Income tax

    Other insurances
    Life, house, car
    National Insurance contributions
    Pensions and sickness fund contributions

    House
    Community Charge and water rates
    Rent or mortgage repayments
    Heating, lighting, telephone, garden

    Food
    At home or outside

    Clothes

    Travel (to work or leisure)
    Public transport, car

    Recreation and education
    (eg newspapers, TV, cinema)

    Personal
    (eg hairdresser, cleaning, laundry)

    Churches and charities

    Other items
    (eg gifts, weddings, birthdays etc)

    TOTAL EXPENSES:

Planning your retirement budget: a checklist

Complete the following budget sheet to compare present income and expenditure with what your expected retirement budget will be.

	Year before retirement £	*Year after retirement* £
INCOME		
Wages/salary (including part-time earnings)		
State retirement pension (and graduated pension)		
Occupational pension		
Other income (eg investment, interest, etc)		
TOTAL INCOME (gross)		
EXPENDITURE		
Income tax		
Other insurances		
Life, house, car		
National Insurance contributions		
Pensions and sickness fund contributions		
House		
Community Charge and water rates		
Rent or mortgage repayments		
Heating, lighting, telephone, garden		
Food		
At home or outside		
Clothes		
Travel (to work or leisure)		
Public transport, car		
Recreation and education		
(eg newspapers, TV, cinema)		
Personal		
(eg hairdresser, cleaning, laundry)		
Churches and charities		
Other items		
(eg gifts, weddings, birthdays etc)		
TOTAL EXPENSES:		

Goal setting and health

1. In goal setting, realistic and specific targets need to be set.

   In setting these goals, take the following into account:

   a) What do I want to achieve concerning my health?
   b) What steps will I take to achieve this?
   c) What resources/support do I need and from where?

2. Now write in the details for changes you will aim to make in:

   a) two weeks

   b) one month

   c) three months

   d) six months

   e) twelve months

I feel . . . will you?

1. A helpful, simple set of phrases has been developed to support people in saying how they feel without accusing or blaming someone else. If a comment is critical it usually produces a hostile or defensive response.

   The phrases which have been found helpful are:

   a) When you did/said .... (an action)
   b) I felt .... (an emotion)
   c) because I thought .... (a thought)

   then

   d) Will you ....? (a specific question requiring a direct answer)

2. **Example** (related to the Wyldes case study)

   Mary says to Jack that she wants to continue working.
   Jack would then say, using the phrases above:

   When you *said you wanted to continue to work*
   I felt *disappointed* (or angry or unhappy etc)
   because I thought *we'd spend more time together*
   and possibly
   Will you *help me with Mother's shopping on Tuesday?*

3. Some care needs to be taken with the words added to these phrases:

   a) A 'you' added after the word 'because I thought' can make the statement sound or actually be blaming or accusing.
   Try the different versions for yourself and see how they sound and the feelings they produce.

   b) If you use part (d) 'Will you . . .' of the phrase, be prepared for a 'No' in reply. An aspect of looking after oneself is:

   i)   Not to ask for something which is impossible;

   ii) To prepare oneself for a 'No';

   iii) To consider what other options and choices there are.

Participants' evaluation form

Name .... Date ....

Programme title ....

Topic(s) covered ....

For items 1 to 5 please CIRCLE , the number in the column which best describes how you feel overall about the programme in terms of

	EXCELLENT	GOOD	FAIR	POOR
1. how **informative** it was	1	2	3	4
2. how **interesting** it was	1	2	3	4
3. how **valuable** it was	1	2	3	4
4. how material was **presented**	1	2	3	4
5. how **well organised** it was	1	2	3	4

For items 6 to 11 please TICK the relevant answers and write in explanations as needed.

6. What in particular have you gained from this programme?

7. How involved have you felt?

not involved enough ☐   about right ☐   too involved ☐

8. How comfortable have you felt about asking questions if you needed an explanation?

very comfortable ☐   OK ☐   Uncomfortable ☐   I had nothing to ask ☐

9. The things **I liked most** about the programme were ....

10. The things I **liked least** about the programme were ....

11. How would you improve the programme for other people looking ahead to retirement?

12. Any other comments.

© CHRE 1991

Appendix 1: Notes on Marketing

Marketing is an important element of establishing and implementing a pre-retirement programme. It may be the responsibility of adult education tutors, course organisers, welfare personnel and staff development officers among others.

Marketing this preparation for retirement approach will involve the use of a number of strategies: developing the right product, for the right people, at the right price, in the right place and at the right time.

Product

The pre-retirement programme in this book has been developed specifically to respond to and meet the needs of people looking ahead to their retirement. As already indicated, the programme has been tested and found to work with a wide range of people.

Describing the product

The Coping with Change model is a unique programme which assists in the development of an individual's life skills in planning and problem-solving, in building confidence and in raising self-esteem; tutors who have used this model of pre-retirement education are encouraged by their observations that:

- the programme raises awareness of issues and concerns, providing the facility for coping with these changes
- participants feel more positive and look forward to their retirement
- participants develop a greater understanding of themselves and their circumstances
- participants feel better able to cope, manage and influence their own future
- participants recognise the number of options and choices they can make in retirement, for example, in the use of their time, in developing new interests and in maintaining or starting new relationships.

Most important, participation in the programme encourages and develops an individual's self-confidence and feeling of self-worth.

This approach therefore has many advantages over the more traditional pre-retirement programme which involves speakers on set topics.

The Target Groups

The target groups may include employers, employees and the local community. This depends largely on where the preparation for retirement programme is being organised.

If the pre-retirement programme is being arranged for a particular organisation, the target group will probably include employees and possibly their line managers.

Alternatively, if the programme is being offered more widely, the target groups will probably include employers and employees from a range of organisations and the local community.

1. Target group - employers

Before approaching an employer it may be helpful to identify the following information concerning the organisation.

What is the policy and practice of the organisation?
What are the attitudes and interests of the employer to preparation for retirement?
What are the attitudes and interests of the employee to preparation for retirement?
How can the employer become engaged with pre-retirement planning?

Which of the following approaches will be most effective to engage employer interest?

    letter
    brochure/leaflet
    telephone call
    appointment/visit
    presentation
    contacts at other levels in the organisation
    recommendations from:
        other employers
        employees
    research/evaluation reports

What is the most appropriate content for each of the selected approach(es)?

Benefits to the company

- seen as good employer
- encourages good employer/employee relations
- develops good community relations
- makes company equal to or ahead of competitors
- more satisfied workforce
- part of staff recruitment package.

Benefits to the employees

- employees learn to manage change more effectively in and out of paid employment
- employees gain a sense of control
- employees learn to understand their own needs
- employees learn to see a more positive future
- employees learn to recognise the caring aspects of the employer.

Publicity to the employer

- Identify employer networks, eg Chambers of Commerce, Rotary Clubs, Lions Clubs etc.
- Identify key manager within an organisation, eg personnel, training, welfare or other relevant senior officer.
- Decide which approach or combination of approaches is required.

Contact the employer in the preferred way.

Send personalised letters to appropriate officers in organisations, followed up by telephone calls and personal visits. Enclose a marketing leaflet and programme plan. Design an attractive brochure/leaflet and be prepared to discuss the costs with any potential 'clients'.

Be aware that negative attitudes exist towards the word 'retirement', therefore other words may be helpful in marketing to the target groups.

Follow-up

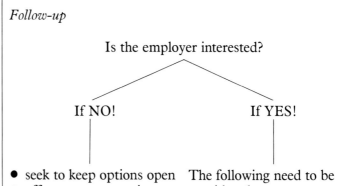

Is the employer interested?

If NO!

- seek to keep options open
- offer to contact again
- provide feedback from other retirement programmes.

If YES!

The following need to be considered:

What will be the type of pre-retirement programme? How negotiable is this? At what ages/stages will employees be involved? What support is available from the employer in terms of?

- recruitment
- publicity
- time off
- staff allocated to provide support, eg personnel or training
- venue/location of event(s), refreshments etc.

2. Target group – potential participants

The best approach to the target group will depend on a number of factors:

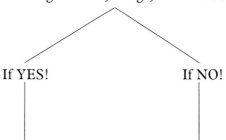

Do they all come from the same community, i.e. the same organisation, village, club or association?

If YES!

If NO!

The ways of reaching the group are relatively more straightforward, and may include such options as:

- in-house newsletter
- memos to members
- letters from key officers
- committee agenda items
- personal recommendations.

If the participants come from a variety of places a wider range of approaches must be used. These may include:

- articles/adverts in local papers, local newssheets, eg Parish news, residents' associations, ethnic newssheets, community centre news etc.
- radio – local news items, what's on, current affairs linked with the place of older people in the community
- adult education brochures
- mailshots/enclosures in local newssheets
- poster advertising
- letters of invitation (see page 125)
- posters in GPs' surgeries, dentists' waiting rooms, libraries, sports centres, banks, social clubs, Citizens' Advice Bureaux.

Remember to include the following points:

Type of programme
Dates and times of the programme
Venue
Costs.

Draft of a 4-page leaflet for employers

Page 1

Title of programme

Possible titles

Coping with change: Focus on retirement
Planning for the future: what do you and your employees need in retirement?
What next? Staff in your organisation
Staff in your organisation – mid and later life planning
Towards the third age: retirement planning
Life span planning
Later life planning
Life long planning
Planning for your future

Organisation

Page 2

Contents

Why plan for the future?

In these times of rapid change in the work, home and social environments, planning for the future is important because it gives people a sense of control, of being in charge of their lives. Recent evidence demonstrates that if we prepare for changes, we understand them better and manage/cope with them more effectively.

What kind of programme is being offered?

A unique programme has been designed around the coping/managing change model.

This programme combines essential aspects of theory and practice to help people to prepare for changes in their future lives. The model considers each course member individually as having distinctive needs and experiences. The programme evolves around the individual, encouraging the sharing of knowledge and experience with other participants.

What are the benefits of this approach to the organisation?

- good publicity and public relations
- the encouragement of good working relationships
- part of the staff recruitment and retention package

Page 3

Is this Coping with Change model effective?

Field tests show that participants:

- feel more positive and look forward to their retirement
- develop a greater understanding of themselves and their situation
- feel better able to cope, manage and influence their own future
- recognise the number of options and choices they have in retirement in the use of, for example, their time, in developing new interests and in maintaining or starting new relationships.

Most important, participation in the programme encourages and develops an individual's self-confidence and feeling of self-worth.

What will it cost?

a) staff time – preparation/teaching
b) resources – materials for participants, audio-visual
c) possible costs of hiring venue and refreshments (detailed by yourselves)

Page 4

> **Include background information about your organisation and its experience**

Publicity – draft letter to employers

(headed paper)

(date)

(Address of employer)

Dear (personalise if possible)

Re ... (title of course or programme)

In times of rapid, and sometimes unexpected, change in the work environment, an increasing number of employers are providing individual counselling and/or pre-retirement/mid-life courses (delete as required) for their employees.

The enclosed leaflet describes the services we can offer to you in this area. In particular we are able to arrange a programme which is relevant for your employees based on the results of a three-year action-research project funded by the Health Education Authority.

The benefit to you, as an employer, could be seen as:
- a contribution to your caring role
- good working relationships
- your employees' ability to manage organisational and personal changes more effectively.

The benefits to your employees could be seen as a contribution to:
- their own abilities in managing organisational and personal change
- a greater understanding of their own attitudes towards change
- the adoption of a positive attitude in both the present and future changes they may meet.

The cost of the programme will be ... (estimate to include hire of venue, resources, staff time). I will telephone your office on .... in the hope of arranging a meeting in the near future.

Yours sincerely

(name)
(institution)

Publicity – draft letter to potential participants

(headed paper)

(date)

(Address of potential participant)

Dear (personalise if possible)

You (and your partner) are invited to a . . . . course on . . . . (date) at . . . . (venue) from . . . . (time) to . . . . (time).

This course has been specifically designed for people approaching retirement, and is based on the results of research which has been undertaken in this area for a number of years.

The whole course is focused on retirement as one of life's important changes, and on the ways we approach this period of life in the 1990s. In a friendly and informal atmosphere we shall consider such questions as 'What does retirement mean to us? How well prepared do we feel for this new phase in life? What information or sources of information do we need to help us at this time? How good are we at managing or coping with life's changes? Are there still things we can learn to help us in the decisions about how we see our lives in retirement?'

The course will be organised and run by experienced staff (tutors) and there will be plenty of relevant literature, addresses of local and national sources of information, etc.

The cost will be . . . . for the . . . . days, and will include (mention accommodation, meals, light refreshments, as appropriate). Please complete the attached reply slip and return it to me by . . . .

Yours sincerely,

(name)
(institution)

Reply slip

To . . . .
Please reserve me . . . . places on the pre-retirement course at . . . . on . . . .
I enclose . . . . (cheque amount) to cover the costs involved.
Name . . . .
Address . . . . .Telephone no . . . .

Appendix 2: Developing the Work

These notes are intended for the more experienced tutor, who has already worked through the Coping with Change model with a group more than once, and is prepared to consider ways in which the work, and possibly his or her own knowledge and skills, might be developed further. Evaluation and assessment, both of personal and group experience, along the lines suggested in the resource materials is most important, but having gone through that process two or three times, the tutor may well be wondering 'What happens next?'

Did the questions which were addressed in the final session (Stages 10–12) give the tutor any general insight into the way in which improvements might be made, or have they simply mirrored the opinions of a few people or even one person?

To what extent did the participants assess the significance of their own participation and involvement? Did they seem to think that the tutor had a hidden agenda, held most of the power and made all the decisions – while they collaborated, albeit quite willingly, with this situation?

In the light of the participants' observations and his or her own reflections, we would encourage the tutor to consider three possible ways of developing this work. First, there is the area of his or her own self-development. Here the intention is to promote further consideration of some of the fundamental questions raised earlier in the text, such as:

- *What is the model trying to achieve?* (i.e. What is the pre-retirement course all about; its aims and content?)
- *What methods are being used?* (i.e. Why are certain techniques advocated, and what personal skills do they bring into use?)
- *Did the tutor feel comfortable with the work?* (i.e. What is the tutor's attitude to the task and the group?)
- *How else might the aims have been achieved?* (i.e. What went well, which parts not so well?)

These questions are directly related to the resource materials – to the use of discussion in small groups, especially at the beginning of the course (Stages 1–4), to the treatment of the ideas of transition (Stages 5–7), to the importance of encouraging involvement and participation in deciding the issues to be looked at (Stages 8 and 9), and to how these issues may best be treated (the four 'themes' of change).

Second, as was explained earlier, these resource materials were originally designed to be used in training courses for tutors who were interested in moving into the field of pre-retirement education. While much of the material may lend itself to staff training/development programmes, this is not the prime aim. However, much 'training' in pre-retirement education goes on in ad hoc ways, such as observing a colleague in action, or 'sitting by Nellie' as it is often described. By offering this opportunity for tutors to consider their own self-development in this work, it is hoped that some practising tutors will be encouraged to invite colleagues to share these experiences of using the Coping with Change approach and so contribute to the wider development of the work.

And third, the Coping with Change model is not limited to preparing for retirement. On the contrary, its application to other times of change in life, such as early retirement, redundancy, returning to work, moving home, becoming a parent, beginning or ending a personal relationship will become more evident the more the model is applied. It is hoped that some tutors will be encouraged to experiment in using this approach with other groups and in other situations.

Working with Groups

In the resource materials we put great emphasis on group work, and lay stress on the value of discussion. As John Stuart Mill said in his essay *On Liberty* (1859):

'There must be discussion to show how experience is to be interpreted . . . The only way a human being can make some approach to the whole of a subject is by hearing what can be said about it by persons of every variety of opinion, and studying all modes in which it can be looked at by every character of mind'

There are several sections in the foregoing text on how to encourage discussion (see pages 14–15 and 42–44). The more experienced tutor may like to reflect further on why preference is given to this method of learning and what its use entails.

Forming a pre-retirement group

In setting up a new course, a tutor usually has very little time to contact participants beforehand, and is often handed a list of names of the course participants shortly before the first meeting. But still, even at this stage, however close to the first meeting, the process of encouraging the separate individuals to start thinking and preparing themselves as members of a particular group, meeting for an agreed purpose, can begin. Hence the importance of the letter of invitation, the way it is written and the indication it gives of the purpose of the course and the method or methods to be adopted (see page 125).

We then suggest a series of practical steps which the tutor may or may not choose to adopt. These include, for instance, attention to seating arrangements and use of name badges (see pages 32–33), and the 'ice-breaking' exercises (Stages 1 and 2) designed to ensure that each participant meets and speaks with all the others early on in the proceedings, and the statements from the tutor, explaining what is being done and why. The key is to create a supportive atmosphere in which participants will feel able to analyse the issues important to them and to talk about their hopes and fears to the extent they decide.

Why the emphasis on group work?

Having gone to the trouble of forming a large group from a number of individuals who may or may not know each other in advance, why then go to the further effort of breaking that group down into smaller groups? In effect, the tutor is adopting a more adult or andragogical (as opposed to pedagogical) approach to learning. While pedagogy is related specifically to the teaching of children, the name 'andragogy' (first used in 1833 by a German grammar school teacher, Alexander Kapp, to describe the education theory of the Greek philosopher Plato) is derived from a combination of the classical Greek agoge (the activity of leading) with the stem 'andr-' (adult).

Theories about andragogy (see, for instance the writings of Malcolm Knowles, 1978) and how it differs from pedagogy are based on four main assumptions:

- *self concept*
  A child is a largely dependent person growing towards autonomy. An adult has achieved psychological maturity.
- *experience*
  Children are relatively new to life's experiences, while adults have accumulated vast quantities of experience of differing kinds
- *readiness to learn*
  With children the teacher decides both the content and the method of learning; while with adults the learners decide with the tutor what it is they wish to learn.
- *time perspective and orientation to learning*
  With children education is perceived as 'preparation for the future', while with adults learning is 'problem-centred' rather than 'subject-centred'. To discover 'where we are now' and 'where we want to go' is the heart of the andragogical approach to education.

Other writers, such as Faure (1972),Gagne (1977), Illich (1973), Jarvis (1983), Kidd (1973), Rogers (1969) and Tough

(1971) all add a great richness to the study of adults learning. While Knowles particularly emphasises the andragogical approach, all the other writers point out that adults bring enormous experience to their learning: that they are free agents in their choice of what to learn: are capable of learning new knowledge at any age, and all these attributes should be taken into account by those who teach them. Hence the value of discussion in the learning process, and its effective use through small group work.

Some questions about the method

What is the optimum size for the small group? How small is small? Are people going to keep to the suggested subject? How will the tutor discover what the groups are really discussing? Will the participants feel resentful, and think they are being denied possibly valuable information or a variety of views which other participants have? Who is in control in each group? Are the same people monopolising leadership roles? Are the participants developing relationships that will help or hinder the course work?

Tutors will develop their own answers to these questions as they observe the groups at work and take note of the feedback they receive. We offer some comments from our own experience.

(1) We have found the most effective small group usually consists of four to eight people. Any number below four is generally too limiting, while more than eight may inhibit the less vocal members of the group.

(2) It is counter-productive to set up discussion groups unless there is a clear reason for doing so. It is also incumbent on the tutor to ensure that the participants have some knowledge of the subject under discussion. Take, for instance, Stage 3 of the resource material – the question 'What does retirement mean to you?' First, the question is phrased in such a way as to seek opinions, and it is fair to assume that everyone attending a pre-retirement course will hold an opinion on that question. Second, if the tutor clearly explains that one of the reasons for discussing this in small groups is to encourage every participant both to listen and to speak, if they wish, then that may be seen as a polite invitation to every participant to be conscious of the value of each contribution.

(3) The tutor needs to keep all the groups under observation. On occasion, it may be necessary to interrupt the proceedings with a general announcement, for example 'We agreed to stop in ten minutes – do try to ensure that everyone has had an equal amount of time to contribute – it may be time to begin your group summary if you haven't already started'. Inviting each group to present a summary of their discussion on a flipchart (or some similar method) enables all

participants to share – and question or clarify – the total experience.

(4) Time is an element common to all groups. It is sometimes maintained that a period of contact time is necessary before the participants involved can become a group. It is important to think about how a close working relationship can best be developed. Some tutors like to formalise the process and agree 'ground rules' with the groups, others simply invite the participants to consider their involvement in the group as an extended informal conversation, such as might take place in their sitting rooms at home.

(5) Inviting participants to work in small groups is no guarantee of a successful session. The most obvious pitfall for the tutor to avoid is inadequate preparation for the task. If the groundwork is thoroughly done, if all the participants understand the reasons for working in small groups and know what they have to do, and understand that their discussion will contribute to the progress of the whole programme, then our experience is that most adults enjoy the experience. If however participants are simply 'told' to 'work in groups', then enormous frustration can build up. People may feel that they are being manipulated, made to play childish games, invited to share each other's ignorance.

Alternative methods

Among other clusters of questions which the tutor may wish to consider further in relation to group work are those which concern his or her personal feelings about the method, professional competence, and of course possible 'failure'. Comparing notes and listening to the experiences of other tutors can be valuable, especially if there is an honest assessment of the measure of success both for the group under scrutiny and for the tutor. In these resource materials we have advised that the less experienced tutor should follow the suggested method, but we are aware that for the more experienced tutor this can hinder rather than promote success. The more confident will make adjustments to suit their own style. There is no substitute for practice.

We would encourage the experienced tutor to consider whether other methods might not be more effective for the particular task in hand. One way of doing this is for the tutor to put himself or herself in the role of the participant, to imagine being a member of a pre-retirement course. Take again Stage 3, and think about how the question, 'what does retirement mean to you?' is treated. If you were a participant, would you prefer to submit an individual written response? Or would you want to respond to an open question to the whole group? Would visual or aural teaching aids stimulate you to more meaningful discussion? What other ways can you suggest? Different tutors will select different methods as most appropriate for that particular task. No one method should be slavishly adhered to unless the tutor and the whole group is confident that it is achieving its aim.

It can be a salutary, exciting and challenging experience for any tutor to evaluate the progress of their own professional skill and knowledge and ask: 'If I decide to use small group work as the most appropriate teaching method for a particular task, what do I bring to the work? Where do I feel there are gaps in my knowledge and skills? What resources do I have to draw on? What is my attitude towards my own development in this aspect of working with adults? Where can I get the help or support I feel I need?'

Managing Change

In the resource materials we frequently refer to the course which we are outlining as the Coping with Change model. Retirement is seen, essentially, as one of life's major changes, and the course focuses particularly on the importance of creating more meaningful understanding both of retirement and of life's changes.

In 1967, two psychologists, Holmes and Rahe, published a table in which they listed 43 life events according to the amount of stress they brought to the individual. The first ten in the order of ranking were:

1. Death of a spouse
2. Divorce
3. Marital separation
4. Jail sentence
5. Death of a close family member
6. Personal injury or illness
7. Marriage
8. Dismissed at work
9. Marital reconciliation
10. Retirement

Retirement, then, is considered to be quite a stressful event. However, it is important to note that the life event of marriage – which presumably is a very happy time for most people – comes higher on the stress-inducing scale than retirement. There is no indication if the writers considered retirement as a happy or sad life event. It is the actual change which has occurred which causes stress, regardless of whether the change is for better or for worse. The level of stress involved, and the ability of the individual to cope with or manage that stress, as we know from everyday events in life, depends on many factors among which is the individual's own attitude to the coming event.

The process of retirement

If Holmes and Rahe were compiling such a list today, it would be interesting to see if retirement still maintained its tenth position. During the last 25 years, as we noted earlier, there have been significant demographic changes. Fewer men are staying in full-time employment until the statutory age of retirement. At the same time more women are taking up full or part-time employment in mid and later life. The timing and nature of that change in life called retirement has itself changed and is still in the process of change. This process is bound to continue as long as retirement is inextricably linked with paid work.

A more detailed look at the work of Stanley Parker to which we referred on page 4, can give us a helpful insight into the meaning of retirement. Parker distinguished three different connotations for 'retirement':

- First, it is an event in life, the date or day of which is known in advance;
- Second, it is a process, indicating a period of time for adjustment from one role (or status) in life to another;
- Third, it is that phase in life when people see themselves as 'retired' and are recognised as such.

The first and third points in his analysis are quite straightforward and easy to accept. The second point is far more complex, for it introduces the notion that a period of time (unspecified) will elapse between the first and third stages during which the person is 'in transition from having paid work to no paid work. This process is encouraged, facilitated – and in a few cases averted – by what various bodies do. The government decides at what age and in what circumstances state pensions shall be payable. The employer has a policy for the retirement of workers, which may take place with or without an occupational pension, when they reach a certain age, in some other circumstances, or not at all'. It is often during this period of transition that a pre-retirement course is held, the purpose of which is usually described as offering help, support and information for people approaching retirement.

Another writer quoted earlier, Colin Murray Parkes, pointed out that 'Human beings are seldom surprised, but their ability to anticipate important changes in their lives enables them to make the necessary changes in their expectations in advance, and *to experience a part of the emotion appropriate to the event before it occurs* [our italics]'. On this basis an important factor in preparation for retirement is to help people to understand the reactions they will experience during the process of retirement. Looking back, many people cannot readily identify when they first thought of their own retirement; Parkes suggests that one of the main reasons people are able to anticipate a part of the emotion appropriate to impending change is that they engage in what he describes as 'worry work'. His emphasis is on 'anticipation', implying that not every change necessarily causes or sets up a cycle of 'worry', and he concludes that 'any plan for change should include an attempt to understand and provide for the psycho-social effects of the change.'

Doubts and difficulties

To what extent can the tutor – usually a younger person than those attending the course – understand the process that the participants are experiencing? As people are individuals and manage or cope with life's changes in their own particular ways, what is so different about retirement? What special knowledge if any does the tutor need to 'teach' people approaching this major change? To what extent can the tutor feel justified in and capable of preparing a course which will create the type of atmosphere within which the participants will feel confident about exploring their feelings as they approach retirement? Where are the parameters, boundaries or guidelines? What happens if the tutor loses control of the situation? These are genuine difficulties, but we can offer some reassurances based on our experiences with training tutors to take pre-retirement groups.

(1) Most tutors have more to offer than perhaps they realise. Some tutors will have experience in personnel work and counselling, for instance. Some may have qualifications in, for example, the field of psychology or sociology. Others will have special knowledge or experience which enables them to take a particular stance on certain issues – health, perhaps, or financial matters. Many will be familiar with the techniques of adult education in other contexts. In general, the approach or attitude to the participants is as important as the knowledge and skills being brought to the task. As both knowledge and skill develop and grow with experience, so too attitudes will change and this will be reflected in the work.

(2) However, irrespective of how the tutor relates to the group, a working knowledge and understanding of life's changes and patterns of transition is essential. Much of this knowledge is quite literally common sense, for all adults must have experienced many changes in their lives. The particular focus for the groups using these resource materials is on retirement – the task for the future is to create that greater understanding of the process of transition which the participants are living through and possibly trying to cope with at their present ages and stages in life.

(3) The pre-retirement course is often seen as a form of intervention in people's lives. The tutor may well wonder

what jusitification he or she might have for intervening, what kind of responsibility is being assumed. Surely this kind of intervention should be the province of some kind of specialist? But tutors should not feel that they are the only source of help and advice. Research shows that people regard professional expertise as only one of several sources of help, and frequently the source of last resort (see, for example, Sugarman, 1986: 'There is substantial evidence that most people first draw upon their own resources and those of kith and kin before approaching official sources of assistance'). And Golan (1981) identified five potential sources of assistance available to a person in need: the self; the natural help system (family, friends, neighbours); the mutual help system (both formal and informal); the 'non-professional' support system (and para-professionals, including voluntary organisations); the professional help system (people with recognised professional qualifications). The pre-retirement tutor is most frequently found amongst the professionals or para-professionals, which means, on the basis of Sugarman's statement, that generally speaking people may have assistance from at least three other sources in evaluating what the tutor says.

(4) There are particular implications for the tutor in recognising the extent to which course participants rely largely on their own abilities and initiatives to cope with change and themselves decide when to extend their contacts to include the natural and mutual help systems. However there is little doubt that few people have received any education to increase their understanding of change and transition. All they know is what they themselves have experienced, from living through their own particular transitions. This lack of a more generalised understanding can lead to feelings of guilt or inadequacy. When we have been introducing the transition curve, for instance, we have often heard participants say 'That is just how I feel – I didn't think other people were also experiencing similar thoughts and feelings – I thought it was only me.' The tutor does have to be sure that the participants understand the experience of transition before they begin the process of planning.

A positive approach

The tutor should be particularly wary of giving the impression that retirement is full of 'problems' which have to be 'solved'. Remember that the idea of 'Coping with Change' found its beginnings in relation to the management of stress. There was from the start an assumption that there was *always* a problem to be solved. The balance is slowly being redressed as people accept that many changes in life are to be welcomed and are developmental in their nature. It should not be assumed that all people approaching retirement foresee a problem-loaded period. On the contrary, many people welcome the approach of retirement and view it very positively. As Danish and D'Augelli (1980) put it: 'As life events are viewed from the developmental perspective as potentially having both positive and negative outcomes, the goal (or aim) of intervention is not the prevention of the critical life per se, but the enhancement of the individual's ability to grow or develop as a result of the event'.

Given the situation in which pre-retirement tutors find themselves, with scant knowledge of the course participants, it may be prudent to explore the understanding of retirement and change with the group to the level of mutual understanding, primarily in order that each participant is able to accept that their feelings about their approaching retirement are both healthy and natural. Point out that the indicators on the transition graph in the resource materials go up as well as down. Emphasise that periods of transition, whether welcomed or feared, usually contain elements of opportunity as well as of risk. The Chinese symbol for 'crisis' has two parts – one meaning danger and the other opportunity. The danger in retirement is inability to cope, while the opportunity is for personal growth. The pre-retirement tutor setting out the aims for the course should find that both helpful and reassuring.

Involvement and Participation

Stages 8 and 9 of the resource materials are designed to involve participants in setting the agenda for the remainder of the course. First, participants review the changes they expect in retirement, and then the various types of change they list are clustered together to form 'themes'. The intention is to enable participants to take and to accept (in Knowles's terminology) some measure of responsibility for their own learning.

Risks and rewards

Where does this leave the tutor? Why embark on a process of learning which may lead to areas hitherto unexplored of which the tutor may have little knowledge? We freely admit that participation in agenda setting does involve such risks (if the tutor chooses to interpret them as such); it is a challenge for all participants, as well as the tutor. But we are convinced that the rewards make the effort involved worthwhile.

(1) By involving all the participants and encouraging them to contribute, the tutor is giving a clear signal that the content or agenda or whatever terms are used which follows after this discussion will reflect the main interests of all the participants. From the participants' point of view, it is also an

acknowledgement that they are being encouraged to be active as opposed to passive learners.

(2) It is also important to recognise that by harnessing the collective experience and interest of all the participants, a measure of both self and group discipline must follow. For example, in listing the changes which will occur at retirement, how is it possible to balance the amount of time which should be given to one major theme of change, such as Finance, with a minority interest such as the compulsory move consequent on having to leave a tied property? After all, the theme of Finance interests the majority of the group, while the theme of Moving Home may possibly be the concern of only one participant. The group will see the inherent difficulty of recognising the issues important for all the participants, whilst also respecting individual aims concerning the quality of each particular life in retirement and will react accordingly.

(3) It is also important to be clear about the amount of time which it is possible to allocate to this agenda-setting exercise and exactly what the participants are expected to do in their groups. As always, the tutor encourages the efficient working of the small groups by careful introduction of the topic. There are two stages to the task: first, to identify those changes that *will* occur to everyone in retirement; and, second, those that *may* occur. These are separate tasks which should impose a structure and a time-frame on the group's deliberations. The purpose is not to analyse the details of the type or number of changes which retirement will or may bring, or to seek a variety of opinions on such detail. Rather it is to prepare an agreed agenda and consider the relevant importance of each item in relation to the expressed needs/ opinions of the participants within a given time-scale. It follows that the tutor needs to be, perhaps, more aware of how each small group is getting on with these functional or practical tasks than on other occasions when the tutor's prime aim in the small group work is to develop a caring, trusting and supportive unit.

(4) When the small groups have completed the agreed task, and go on, in Stage 9, to share the results of their deliberations, then clearly a new stage in the process begins. The bringing together, or clustering, of the issues raised by the participants creates the opportunity for the whole group (including the tutor) to clarify such points as the actual meanings or interpretations of the words being used in the clusters and of the relative importance and emphasis given to the various aspects of a theme. For instance, the general theme Finance may include matters such as 'making a will', or 'investing a lump sum of money' as well as 'managing a weekly budget on a reduced income' or prioritising what may be described as essential as opposed to optional spending. It is

important to emphasise that none of these matters is actually being discussed at this stage, but having them highlighted enables participants to prepare for the next step in the process of coping with the change in the context of finance. It also encourages participants to reflect on the stage in transition they have reached at this particular time.

Alternative approaches

Having used the approach suggested in the resource materials of arriving at an agreed agenda by encouraging the active involvement of all the participants, the tutor may like to consider different ways which are often used to achieve the same objective.

It is of course possible to involve adult students in course planning through the use of questionnaires, through individual consultations or through meeting the whole group in pre-course sessions. Very occasionally pre-retirement courses are advertised as 'open-discussion' – a few employers offer such courses which usually consist of a one-day meeting on a monthly basis over a period of a year. This gives a total of twelve meetings of seven hours, equal to a total course time of some 84 hours. Most pre-retirement tutors would consider that provision as sheer luxury for during the 84 hours all the issues and topics identified by the participants can be included, and there is still time enough between each meeting for reflection to take place, information to be gathered and advice to be sought on specific topics of personal interest to the participants.

In a typical pre-retirement course, we acknowledge that all participants are different and will expect different things from the course. But it is the tutor who plays the crucial role in setting out realistic aims and in determining the appropriateness of the methods used in achieving them. Much depends on the tutor's skill, experience and self-confidence. However, it is worth repeating that research into how, why and in what circumstances adults learn most effectively clearly indicates that the key factor is the motivation of the learners and their perceptions as to the relevance of the knowledge they gain. Therefore one of the most important tasks for the tutor in pre-retirement education is constantly to seek out the content appropriate for the particular group in order to produce an efficient and effective programme. This aim, whether achieved or not, makes all the background reading and course preparation worth the effort.

Themes of Change

In the resource materials we have distinguished four main 'themes of change' which we have found are usually areas of concern for people approaching retirement. Although they are treated separately in the text, there is no reason why any one theme should either precede or take precedence over another. For example, the first theme discussed in the text is Time – that is to say, the number or cluster of issues which the participants identified round the use of time in retirement. There is universal recognition that the imperatives of paid work on the one hand create a structure for the worker's life whilst, on the other, impose limits on the worker's freedom of choice. Havighurst (1961) actually described retirement as a 'crisis in the meaningful use of time'. People who are approaching retirement are often asked 'What are you going to do when you retire?', as though they are expected to be able to list a number of activities to prove they will be capable of occupying themselves once they are without the structure which paid work has imposed. There seems to be a pressure on the respondent to give a satisfactory reply, as though there were some hidden assessment of personal success or failure; the simple message is that society expects the retired to be able to fill their time usefully. These and other external pressures the participants bring to the course and present a real challenge to the knowledge and skill of the tutor.

Planning for the future

However, the course tutor preparing a session on the use of time will quickly find that it is difficult to separate the issues raised under that heading from other changes which occur at retirement. We know that changes in the structure and use of time, in finance, in relationships and in health will *all* occur at this time. The dilemma facing those approaching retirement and therefore those who prepare pre-retirement programmes is that any division or separation between these changes is purely artificial. These changes are all being experienced – to a greater or lesser degree for each individual – as life is lived during this period of transition.

It is therefore crucial that treatment of each theme focuses on each of the following three steps in the Coping With Change model in turn:

- taking stock;
- identifying issues;
- making choices.

This is the 'planning' stage of the course where a clear understanding of the effects of change in all its many facets will help each participant identify the key issues for him or herself, bring them together, reflect on their relative importance, and thus be in a better position to consider the range of options available and to choose accordingly.

A further shift in the progress of the course can also be detected at this stage. Up to this point great emphasis has been laid on working together, as a whole group or in small discussion groups in order to come to a fuller understanding of what retirement means. Now the tutor begins to encourage each participant to take the responsibility for developing his or her own plans. Here the benefits of forming and working together in small groups should begin to show and each participant should be able to look back at the early beginnings of the course with some satisfaction. In a very practical way it is at this time in particular that he or she may well find their knowledge and experience being widely sought, while at the same time themselves needing similar resources from other members of the group.

A comprehensive approach

So, though in the resource materials we advise the less experienced tutor to begin by separating out clusters of issues into various 'Themes of Change', we recognise that a very strong case can be made for taking a more comprehensive approach. We have included a written case study, The Wyldes (Handout 3a and 3b), which can be used as a basis for discussion of issues around financial planning, health matters and changing relationships as well as in the use of time – or indeed of all these issues together. This combined case-study approach has been used very effectively on a number of courses, especially where time is limited.

Remember, the written case study is a story, and the story can be adapted to reflect the circumstances of the group and its individual members. In thinking about the Wyldes' affairs, participants should be encouraged to consider how the individual characters in the story, such as Jack or Mary or Marion, view their own and each other's retirement, what thoughts may be uppermost in their minds (invent them if they are not in the text), what issues are most important to them and in what ways it can be proposed that they proceed to cope with the changes involved and move and adjust towards successful retirement.

Using a written case study in this instance and looking at the different characters in it in this way, can also often help participants understand how differently men and women may view many of the issues raised. For example, Jack Wylde, in planning what he is going to do in retirement, will find it necessary to consider people other than himself and realise that one of the first steps in his planning would be to talk things through with Mary, his wife. Jack and Mary cannot make meaningful decisions in isolation, and they in turn are affected by what Marion does – and so on. It is surprising how often in real life one partner thinks he or she knows instinctively how the other is thinking and will react, without the need for discussion, only to be proved wrong when an issue is discussed together.

If the tutor decides to use one case study throughout the course, this would have implications for visiting 'experts' (people with special subject knowledge in, for example, finance or health). They could then be invited to take part in the group's activities as consultants, responding to issues which emerged from studying the case. In any briefing session with a visiting 'expert' it would be important for the tutor to include a copy of the case study and a summary of the issues which had emerged in discussion. This approach differs from the usual briefing recommended for visiting experts in that the group discussions will have produced a number of different issues which are interwoven and not clearly listed in one specialist subject area or another. Many visiting experts usually resist making comments on matters they consider to be outside their professional knowledge, but may well be prepared to do so within the context of the case study. This is our experience. Major issues in life are seldom, if ever, neatly compartmentalised, and if it is recognised that there are clear differences between giving factual information and stating opinion then much can be learnt from the professional approach to a problem.

Tutors with experience of using written case studies may prefer to prepare their own, as suggested in the text. Some tutors have extended the method by encouraging participants to develop a group case study. The story starts at the beginning of the course and may be triggered by a photograph or video or an idea from the group member; it develops as the issues emerge and the need for planning becomes imperative.

Irrespective of the method used, it is important that each individual participant considers the task or problem stages of the Coping with Change model and is able to 'practice' and test the routes or options, decision making and other processes in a safe and friendly environment. Some participants may be very skilled and experienced in problem-solving and use methods which they have refined over many years, while others may shy away from the notion of planning and claim that it is more natural for them not to plan. These differences of opinion are extremely valuable within the group for they promote meaningful discussion on individual interpretations of planning as a conscious activity and enable the tutor to demonstrate both the instrumental and flexible nature of the Coping with Change model approach.

Conclusion

Finally, it must be said again that this is a process rather than a content model and the more the tutor designs and operates the same process, the more the course will develop and the more the tutor will acquire that individual reservoir of knowledge and skills.

The inherent temptation of repeating the same process because of one success is as prevalent in a process as in a content model, especially if the tutor is working in a large organisation. Here it may easily be assumed that, because all the course participants work for the same employer their retirement 'agendas' will be the same. Nothing could be further from reality in our experience. Although most groups will readily identify the same changes that will occur at retirement – such as finance, health, relationships, and time – they will not necessarily consider their importance to them in the same hierarchical order nor agree on the emphasis they place on certain features. For example, if there are more women than men in the group, it is quite feasible to forecast that, in view of current legislation and recent pensions practice, interest in personal taxation would be greater than in employer pensions.

However, it does seem extremely difficult for the work of pre-retirement education to develop without the accompanying development in the knowledge, skills and attitudes of the tutorial staff. We would particularly encourage tutors to recognise any signs of change in societal, governmental or individual attitudes towards retirement and consider the most appropriate ways of preparing programmes or working with individuals who find themselves having to cope with these new situations. But the search for new meanings in changing situations often results in ad hoc responses, to the neglect of fundamentals and proven theories. This situation often arises when large numbers of people are declared redundant in mid-life or when massive take-overs of businesses occur. It is at such times of unexpected change that the experienced tutor is most needed. The professionalism of the tutor is rooted as much in his or her theoretical understanding of change as in their teaching skills. To be able to interpret complex theories of change and transition in the context of the situation in question, and to share this understanding with mature adults with humility and with authority, is the hallmark of the empathetic tutor.

Such knowledge can be acquired and such skills can be practised. The tantalising position in this area of work is that there is no set or fixed body of knowledge. Our knowledge increases as we practise using the process model. The frontiers of knowledge are continually being extended, and the novice tutor of today becomes the developmental pioneer, entrepreneur of tomorrow.

We recognise that at present there are few programmes of training and that resources are limited. However, we have suggested some books for further reading in the text and below, and recommend all tutors to use the resource centres at the Health Education Authority, Hamilton House,

Mabledon Place, London WC1SH 9TX and at the Pre-Retirement Association, Nodus Building, University of Surrey, Guildford GU2 5XM where the Centre for Health and Retirement Education (CHRE) is now located.

References

Danish, S.J. and D'Augelli, A.R., quoted in Sugarman, op.cit.

Faure, E. *Learning to Be* UNESCO, Paris, 1972.

Gagne, R.M. *The Conditions of Learning*. Holt, Rinehart and Winston. New York, 1977.

Golan, N., quoted in Sugarman, op.cit.

Holmes, T.H. and Rahe, R.H. 'The social readjustment rating scale', *Journal of Psychosomatic Research*, Vol. II, pp 213–218.

Illich, I, *Deschooling Society*, Penguin Books, Harmondsworth, 1973.

Jarvis, P., *Adult and Continuing Education, Theory and Practice*. Croom Helm, 1983.

Kidd, J.R. *How Adults Learn*, Associated Press. Follett Publishing Co. Chicago, 1973.

Knowles, M.S. *The Adult Learner: A Neglected Species*. Gulf Publishing Co. Houston, 1978.

Rogers, C.R. *Freedom to Learn*, Charles E. Merrill Publishing Co. Ltd, Columbus, Ohio, 1069.

Sugarman, L. *Life-Span Development*, Methuen, 1986.

Tough, A. *The Adult's Learning Projects*, Ontario Institute for Studies in Education, Toronto, 1979.